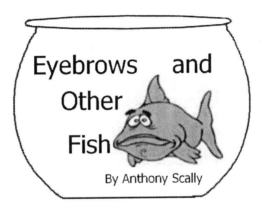

Eyebrows and Other Fish

By Anthony Scally

Apart from my own, some of the mental health professionals and those people already in the public eye, names have been changed.

Over one million people each year commit suicide-World Health organization

Published by

Chipmunkapublishing Ltd

PO Box 6275

Brentwood

Essex CM13 1ZT

United Kingdom

Copyright © 2007 by Anthony Scally

Acknowledgements

Anthony Seaborn my current Support Worker has helped me enormously being my sounding board and giving me feedback. He has supported me throughout and without that support it just would not have happened.

Peter Roberts, Mary Moloney, Professor Shôn Lewis (Adult Psychiatry, University of Manchester), Geoff Woods (Community Psychiatric Nurse), Marion Heyes and Sandor Szabo have all believed in me and this from the start and I owe them all thanks for that.

"Although *Eyebrows and other fish* is written in a colloquial style which you don't often find in printed books, and is at times almost alarmingly honest about aspects of Scally's personal life (and therefore not recommended for anyone with a sensitive disposition), it is an extremely absorbing account of life "with a head full of chaos".

If you want to know what it is like to live with the kind of thought patterns that lead to a diagnosis of schizophrenia, to get a sense of how it feels to be labelled with such a diagnosis, and to get a handle on what it is like to find yourself on the receiving end of the best and worst of mental health services, this is the book to read."

Helen Finch, Mind Publications

Anthony Scally

Contents

Preface

Anthony Scally

Preface

Diabetes
a disease in which the body cannot control the level of sugar in the blood

Diabetic
someone who has diabetes

Schizophrenia
a serious mental illness in which someone cannot understand what is real and what is imaginary: *paranoid schizophrenia*

Schizophrenic
someone who suffers from schizophrenia

Synchronicity
'meaningful coincidence'

(Source: Cambridge Advanced Learners Dictionary 2006)

I don't like labels and 'schizophrenic' does not and should not characterise me, just as diabetic does not personify somebody with diabetes. Schizophrenia is a 'disease' that is not well understood and is greatly feared, and most of what people think they know about schizophrenia is wrong. Unlike diabetes schizophrenia is baffling and controversial, and there are still some intellectuals that are dubious about whether there is a biological basis to it. People confuse schizophrenia with split personality or multiple personality. They also believe that people diagnosed with schizophrenia are violent and dangerous. A limited number are, of course, but media publicity about particularly frightening and bizarre crimes of violence committed by people with mental disorders has left the public with the impression that most people diagnosed are violent. This is simply not true the majority of people diagnosed with schizophrenia are not violent we are all individuals and not the same. If you take any large group of people a small percentage of them may be violent, whether it is football fans, plumbers or even people with diabetes. Schizophrenia has many symptoms but violence is not one of them. Let's not forget that some people are inherently violent and as you might expect some of those people encounter health problems.

The term 'schizophrenia' was introduced in 1911 by a Swiss psychiatrist, Eugen Bleuler. The word comes from the Greek schizo meaning 'split' and phrenia meaning 'mind'. Bleuler wanted to convey the split between what is perceived, what is believed, and what is objectively real. He did not mean that the person with schizophrenia is split into two personalities, but that there is a splitting away of the personality from reality. The concept of 'split', however, has led to schizophrenia being confused with multiple personality, a less common and very different psychiatric disorder, much publicised through stories such as *Dr. Jekyll and Mr. Hyde, The Three Faces of Eve, and Sybil.* Today, many health care professionals regret the existence of the term 'schizophrenia' because of the confusion and misunderstanding that surround it. Then there are those people who believe that people diagnosed with schizophrenia have weak personalities and have 'chosen' their madness. The stigma of schizophrenia is a barrier to those trying to rehabilitate themselves and it is also a very real problem for their families.

Come with me on a journey, this is my experience and everybody's is different. I have had to revisit some unhappier times and it hasn't been easy, not just the writing but the memories it has evoked. We all have experiences we will remember forever, happy and unhappy, serious and comical, and yes I have laughed along the way. How can there ever be anything funny about schizophrenia I hear you cry! Well it's something I live with so it's like asking how can there ever be anything funny in life. If you think of somebody with diabetes again, their life may change somewhat when they are diagnosed but it doesn't change who they are.

Anthony Scally

If you've been diagnosed with schizophrenia or feel you may have it this is important.

There is only one way to read this book and that is the way you are reading it now, nothing subliminal, and there is no code to crack, even if I were that clever I am not that insensitive.

That goes for everyone else too!

Chapter One: Code and conduct

Early June 1990

Electronic Parts Distributor Manchester

Dear Anthony

Further to your interview on Tuesday we are pleased to offer you the position of Full Time Technician with the company. We look forward to seeing you for your first week, starting Monday the 4th. Please telephone Janet the company secretary to confirm.

Yours Faithfully

Dave Greenaway (Manager)

———

I must have read it four or five times this was just marvellous news, it had been several years of being on one scheme or another but this would be my first real job. I went along to lots of different interviews and filled in many application forms and the letter I usually got would be a disappointment and quite soul destroying. I never minded being on the YTS and other schemes but was always disappointed when the promise of a real job at the end of it never happened. I became very cynical about the whole thing thinking where there is a scheme there must be a schemer. I began to think about what it would mean in real terms and obviously the monthly salary would make a big difference. I could buy nice Christmas presents for my daughter and my Mam and I could start to buy things for the flat as well as better food and some new clothes.

I lived in a bed-sit flat in a high-rise block on the 7th floor. I had a kitchen a bathroom and a lounge/bedroom. It was clean and tidy as I have always been a sort of house-proud person. I had managed to get on the phone and had an alarm fitted which was paid for through my electricity slot meter. Funny in a way as it was the money in the meter as to why the alarm was necessary. I owned an electric cooker a fridge and a washing machine. I had a small portable telly that I hardly watched and radio that I hardly ever switched off. I would save for what I needed and sometimes would buy second hand. It usually meant eating cheap noodles or suchlike for a few months.

It was the morning of this letter that I decided to change my ways to include my dope smoking habits and it made perfect sense to me. It was a mixture of boredom and my pursuit of enlightenment that had got me started. Listening to (or appreciating) music whilst stoned was somehow part of my learning or my growing up. I never really got things done whilst stoned though let alone hold down a 9 to 5. I wouldn't say I was a 'stoner' or 'weed head' it was something I did recreationally and actual quantities and frequency were not substantial. One of the problems with it for me was the whole culture of actually getting hold of the cannabis and the loop in which I became caught up in. Another problem was that these days I was not entirely comfortable being stoned feeling somewhat guilty or ashamed and often paranoid.

I went to the drawer in the kitchen where I kept a wooden box no bigger than a small margarine tub. There was a small amount of cannabis resin only enough for two joints at the most. I decided these would be the last two I would ever smoke. I built the two joints and was halfway through the first when I got the 'munchies' (I really needed to eat). It was a Mother Hubbard moment in the kitchen until I spotted the self raising flour that I didn't remember ever buying. Then in the fridge there were eggs and margarine and yes I had sugar. It was going to be very basic but I was going to bake a big cake! A fitting meal of celebration I thought even though it was only 8am.

The cake had been in the oven for about ten minutes or so and I had just extinguished the last ever joint I was going to smoke. The smoke in the lounge was thick and the weed hung heavy in the air. I was feeling quite relaxed when suddenly there was loud banging on my front door. Shit! I hate having to be straight acting whilst stoned so I decided I would ignore it. I could hear some sort of commotion on the landing outside and then the banging again on my door. Shit! Shit! Crap! I left the lounge went down the short hallway and opened the door. A policeman his helmet under his arm walked straight in took three strides down the hallway and into the living area. Be normal pretend you've just woken up I was telling myself as I followed him into my lounge. I stood there saying nothing but rubbed my eyes and faked a half yawn. I managed to kick the ashtray under my bed my heart was thumping as I had visions of being arrested there and then. "We have to evacuate the building young man there's a gas leak two floors below". I thought about crossing the room to open the balcony door but I couldn't look him in the eye. I sat down on the edge of my bed and was pulling on my socks when he turned on what seemed like one heel. I thought he was leaving but he stopped and turned round again. "Best turn everything off, smells lovely by the way". I can only guess the smell he meant was the cake but that is something I shall never know! I was just relieved that I didn't get nicked over my last ever joint.

It wasn't too long before British Gas sorted out the problem on the 5th floor. I decided to take the stairs back up to the flat as there were over 40 other tenants making their way back too. In amongst the used condoms and syringes that littered the stairwell there were dandelions. I thought it odd at the time and wondered if it was meant to mean anything. I had been doing that a lot lately looking for hidden meanings or messages. The smell of urine was almost too much to bear and I found myself holding my breath. In itself it isn't too bad but whilst climbing stairs and still being under the influence of the cannabis it seemed like I would never be home. It was like being on a treadmill as it seemed I was putting in a lot of effort but physically getting nowhere. I could hear some of the other tenants and their doors being banged shut below me. Eventually I reached the flat and once I got inside I opened my balcony door and collapsed onto the bed.

I woke to sounds coming from outside it was the laughter of young children. I was just in time for Radio 4's lunchtime news so I switched the radio on. I went into the kitchen opened the oven and put the cake into the bin the tin as well. The cake had overcooked itself whilst the oven was cooling down and it would have been like chewing a breeze block. I had lost my appetite by now anyway (probably on the stairs). I looked out of my kitchen window down onto the large green area that was to the rear of the block. There were two kids aged about six or seven a boy and a girl they were picking dandelions. I started to think about my daughter Lorna who lives with my Mam Vera. Lorna was seven years old but going on 37 and she is the apple of my eye and always cheerful. I lived with them both for a while but it soon became apparent that Vera had a certain way of bringing Lorna up and that me being there was at odds with that. I would spoil Lorna and would get into arguments with my Mam about it. Lorna didn't help matters any by the usual things kids do in playing one off against the other. The final straw for Vera was the occasion where a teacher had hit Lorna hard on the hand. I went along to the school and made an official complaint. Vera wasn't happy about me doing that and it wasn't too long after that I left leaving Vera to raise Lorna on her own.

It was on the first day of my new job that I realised the title Technician may be overstating my duties. It mainly consisted of me cleaning the warehouse and office space. I was also responsible for changing light bulbs, emptying litter baskets and shredding cardboard. Dave the manager told me that he had some changes planned and my skills in painting and decorating would be put to good use. I had no formal training in painting and decorating but I used to watch my Dad and as I got older would help him. Dave seemed a pleasant friendly character he was not very tall but his height wasn't the first thing I noticed. It was at the initial interview when his eyebrows got my full attention they seemed much darker than his full head of light brown hair. I had decided that their shape was reminiscent of a pair of dolphins that were facing each other and they were animated too!

It was on around the third day that I first met Carmen I was restocking the powdered tea and coffee etc. in the drinks machine. "They got any drinking chocolate yet?" I turned and saw one of the girls from the office a very pretty black girl about my age with big brown eyes and she was very smartly dressed. She put out her hand and I noticed she was wearing a wrist watch that was slightly too big but very feminine with a thin gold strap. I shook her hand limply and she smiled. "Hi, I am Carmen". I looked away and into the box of powdered drinks. "Nope am afraid still no chocolate" I said. "I am Anthony but people here seem to prefer to call me Tony". Still smiling she said, "It's all I will drink". I told her I would speak to Dave about getting some more. "We've all noticed how clean and tidy the place is and how it smells nicer in the toilets". At the risk of sounding forty years old I said, "I do my best". I couldn't help but notice that she had a nice complexion there were no signs of make-up and she also had the most wonderful smile. "It's nice to meet you Tony". She turned and headed back in the direction of the office and I watched her as she walked away. She was stunning what a figure a most wonderful shape. I think it was more of my male programming that made my stare linger than any real wish to know her better besides she was wearing a wedding ring.

There was a freak summer storm that evening it was windy and the rain was coming down heavily in sheets. I was sitting upstairs on the back seat of a double-decker on my way to see my Mam and Lorna. In those days it was like a fog up there as it was the designated smoking area. To be precise it used to be designated for smokers but it was now being discouraged with signs requesting not to. It wasn't policed and there weren't any penalties or fines hence still foggy. I lit my first since leaving work knowing that my stop would be in the next few minutes. I don't think smokers get as much enjoyment from a fag in the outdoors even when it isn't raining. That is probably why we tended to light up on buses and for me it was a case of old habits die hard. I have always used public transport never having learned to drive and I doubt I could even get insurance if I were to pass my test now. The windows were steamed up and I wiped the one nearest to me with the palm of my left hand. I saw the self inflicted tattoos across my fingers - 'MCFC'. I had done them when I was younger whilst in care. I was very self conscious about the tattoos now and would sometimes hide that hand because of it. A Manchester City FC badge would have been much less conspicuous and not as permanent. The rain outside was unrelenting but for now I didn't care. If I am inside or sheltered on a rainy day I always get a certain sense of comfort. I pressed the bell for my stop and made my way downstairs hiding the lit cigarette as I went. I threw the half smoked fag onto the wet pavement and made my way along the street towards the top road. The street on both sides is lined with terraced houses so I made sure I walked well away from the sides of the houses where the guttering needed attention.

I got into my Mam's house and as usual it was warm and welcoming with the telly on in the corner of the room. I put my wet jacket over the radiator and dried my hair with a warm towel I took from the same radiator. Lorna was sat colouring with wax crayons on the floor and Vera appeared from the kitchen with a bowl of stew. I often called her Vera and never Mum because growing up it was always 'Mam'. "Ooh, thanks Vera I am ready for this, any bread?" It was the adverts in the break of Coronation Street and Lorna was singing away to one of the ads. "If yar lark a lorta chocolate on yer biscuit join our club". After eating two bowls of stew and about eight rounds of bread I decided that one more bowl should do it. "Now that I am working Vera if you need anything let me know". I took a packet of cigarettes and a small galaxy chocolate bar from my inside coat pocket. "There's a packet of fags I got for you and it's not a club but I got you a bar of chocolate Lorna". I had bought them out of what I thought was to be my last ever giro cheque. I replaced the coat on the radiator as it still wasn't quite dry. "Not till after her tea" Vera said sternly. "Awe Nana… thank you Dad I prefer these but I have been brainwashed with the club song". I thought about what she had said and what a clever little girl using words like brainwashed and in the right context too. I had finished my third bowl of stew and we were laughing making up a story about the fight in the biscuit tin. 'The Bandit hit the Penguin over the head with a Club and he made a Breakaway in a Taxi…' In the end we must have had a long paragraph worth of biscuit story and it included the 'theft of the Trophy with the Blue Ribbon around it'. The odd sherbet lemon or other such sweet was thrown in by Vera as she never quite got the gist of it bless her but it added to our amusement. It was almost bedtime for Lorna by the time I decided to make my way home. It was dark and the pavements still wet but at least my coat was dry and the wind and rain had stopped.

On the bus going home I noticed some of the adverts that were beginning to appear on the buses. I had a problem with advertising and subliminal messages it had started a few months ago. I started to wonder whether it was simply about the product and getting our money or something more sinister. As if somehow they were there to give those that were 'in the know' instructions or information. I decided that maybe I needed to somehow be 'in the know' so to speak. This was another reason I decided to stop smoking the cannabis when I did because I knew it was a paranoid way of thinking. Anyone who has encountered paranoia as a result of smoking dope knows once the effect of the drug has gone that it was the drug that caused the paranoia. So in effect you knew even before smoking the cannabis that there may be a likelihood of being paranoid. It is a common topic amongst smokers 'being para' or 'getting the paras' however, whilst actually paranoid that insight or knowledge went out of the window for me.

By my third week of work Dave the manager had had me paint and wallpaper the trade counter and two small offices. I had also plastered over a doorway and created a doorway through a hollow plasterboard wall. I had re-glazed a cracked window and on my own initiative cut away the badly stained carpet around the drinks machine. It left a neat concreted area which I painted with grey floor-paint. All this as well as keeping the place clean and tidy.

It was a few days later that Dave was stood at the drinks machine looking down at where I had made the alterations. He turned to me and said, "Can I have a word with you in my office". His dolphins were giving nothing away and I thought crikey I shall offer to pay for the carpet out of my wages. In the office his face lit up with a wide smile "You've been working very hard and we are all pleased with the results what do you know about computers?" Now I didn't want to show my ignorance as I knew very little. I just said something I had heard on the radio. "I thought a megabyte was a big mac". I grinned and he laughed genuinely and loudly. "You see I think you are too good for cleaning and now that the other work is done I would like you to work in sales in the office". The dolphins seemed on calm waters as he outlined his proposal. "It will mean an extra £80 in your wage packet before tax of course". I hadn't even been paid for my first month and already a promotion to say I was pleased was understating it a bit. "It'll be shirt and tie from tomorrow do you have a tie?" I nodded in response and then his two dolphins nodded to one another. It would be good to get out of the boiler suit that was for sure. Just as I was leaving the office he said, "Big mac indeed you're bloody crackers". It seemed an odd word to use 'crackers' not that I knew his vocabulary or anything it just didn't seem to fit with his broad Lancashire accent.

Now the stock (parts) carried by this relatively small company was massive. Everything from diodes, chips, pcb's and capacitors to motors for microwaves and heads for VCR's. There was almost everything you can think of for the inside of most high street makes and models of electronic products. My first two days in the sales office were spent familiarising myself with the operating systems of the computers, the fax machine, telephone system and photocopier. Then it was in at the deep end and if I got stuck put the caller on hold and ask for help, which was something everyone did in the office from time to time. Most of the callers were account holders i.e. service engineers who needed parts to fix microwaves, TV's, hi-fi's, camcorders, VCR's etc. Now and again members of the public would telephone asking for parts but they were charged more as they were non account holders and didn't qualify for trade prices. It was a steep learning curve for me and after a few more days I was dealing with the callers without having to put them on hold. After a few weeks it was me that the others in the office were asking for help. I got to know lots of different part-numbers and stock codes and the makes and model numbers of lots of different appliances. Customers started to ask to be dealt with by me personally and I was really enjoying my time in the office.

The office staff were a small friendly team there were only five of us in all. It was Ian who had been with the firm the longest, he was intelligent but a bit cocky with it. There was Liz a chain smoker who had a grown up son that she never stopped talking about. Peter was bisexual and didn't keep it a secret, his pride and joy was his car which happened to be purple. Then there was Carmen who was quiet and didn't have a lot to say when it came to general office chit-chat. With my first wage I purchased a cheap carpet which I fitted in my main room and I bought a vacuum cleaner. I had started to buy better food with which to stock my cupboards and fridge and ultimately my belly. I always had cigarettes and I hadn't gone back to smoking cannabis, it had been five weeks by now, not that I was counting or even missing it. I had given Vera some money for feeding me for the first few weeks whilst I waited for my wage to go into the bank. I still had money to see me through until the next pay day and it seemed like life was just beginning to turn around for me.

I would always be punctual to work which wasn't a problem as I have always been an early riser. I would normally be up at around 6am each day. On a work day I would usually have a simple breakfast of cereal or toast and occasionally a boiled egg with toast. At weekends I treated myself to the full English. I would sometimes get up earlier than usual and nip across town to see my Mam on workdays. Well, it was to get shirts and pants ironed for work, but it was always good to see her. Ironing is something I can do if I have to but is something I would readily pay to have done. Work started at 8.30am and the bus journey varied between 30 minutes to 45, it was all dependant on traffic. There was about 8 minutes of walking time to and from each bus stop.

On the journeys into work I became preoccupied with car registration plates (number plates). I think it was just to break the monotony of the journey like young children do when they play a spotting game. It started off very simply by just seeing if there were any 'sought after' or 'cherished' plates (number plates that at a glance spell out a name or word). Then as the weeks went by I would try and see if there were any common letters or numbers relating to the colours, makes or models of the vehicles. Now we all know that a car number plate can tell the ordinary person the year the vehicle was manufactured. My trouble was that I believed that it also contained other information too. It seemed certain to me that there must be a sequence or significance of each one. Initially my thoughts were just sarcastic but then they went to being critical about some drivers. All the numbers and letters were giving me headaches so I concentrated on just the colour of the car. If I became 'interested' in a certain car or driver I would make a mental note of the numbers and letters of the plate. I found myself forming all sorts of opinions about the drivers from the colours or plates of their vehicles.

The registration was 'G' that year for new cars and initially I would consider that they must be well off to be driving a G reg car and then I'd wonder what their occupation was. I would sometimes wonder if they had stolen the car! Was it a company car or was it a car on finance and were they married or single. The trouble was it went from me wondering to me assuming or deciding. I would sometimes assume their sexuality or the way they voted and if they used drugs. I was making huge leaps of judgement regarding all sorts of things. I decided that anyone who owned or drove a brown car was not to be trusted, they were sinister or not all they are cracked up to be. I think it was a case of not seeing many brown cars and not being able to get my head around anyone actually wanting or choosing the colour brown. I was so wrapped up in it all it just became something I did without even thinking (oddly though in reality I was thinking far too much).

As the weeks went by this all got ever so intense, the trouble was it went from cars to front doors. Then to ties, shirts or blouses and even socks! All the way along I was still refining the 'code' and hadn't cracked it yet! Was the item worn or was it keeping them safe (like a front door). If it was worn was it upper body or lower. For example somebody who wore green socks was walking on green but green is associated with Ireland. 'They are hangin' people for the wearin' o' the green' I would recall hearing or reading somewhere. If they are walking all over green they were anti-green or were they anti-Irish? A person with a green shirt has it covering their upper body (below the rib cage is the heart and other important organs) was it that they had green in their heart or was green protecting them like some sort of breastplate or shield. Was I even right about what the colour green signified and what did all the other colours signify. For the people who wore yellow I would wonder if it meant they were cowards, obviously if their socks were yellow they didn't like cowardice. The Tories were blue, Labour was red and it was a big year politically for the greens (Green Party) in the European Elections, I really needed to sort this out. It was like a code, dress code, colour code, numbers, letters and combinations. I just knew I needed to get to the bottom of it and get it all straight in my head. I had begun to show even more of an interest in things around me. I decided that Purple cars were driven by people who were bisexual, neither red nor blue but both colours mixed they were sitting on the fence. For the number plates I had mastered what today is known as text speak (or is that txt spk) like in text messages to a mobile phone. C = see, U = you, B = be or in combination: H8 = hate and NE = any, etc. I wasn't sure whether X = women and Y = men, or whether X = ex (as in previous) or Y = why? It tended to be 'useful' for working out certain number plates. To the outside world, my family and colleagues, there was nothing out of the ordinary or unusual about me because nothing had changed. They did not know what I was thinking, how on earth could they, apart from my thoughts I went along with my life in the usual way. At this stage it was my thought processes affecting me and not my behaviour as a result of them. Nobody knew about it and I never knew it was a cause for concern it was something I just did, part of my thinking and I couldn't control the way I thought.

It was during lunch one day in the office that Carmen asked me for a favour. Two people would cover the phones during lunch and it tended to be Carmen and I who did it most days. We usually ate sandwiches or chips at our desks and if a call came through whoever didn't have a mouthful of food would take it. The only call that came through that lunchtime was from Brian, Carmen's husband. I made my way down to the drinks machine and when I returned the office was silent apart from the hum of the photocopier. I was halfway through the remainder of my sandwich when Carmen asked me whether I would be prepared to do some tiling in her kitchen. "Of course we will pay you" she said. To be totally honest the idea didn't appeal to me, although I can do that sort of work I didn't enjoy doing it. I did it for money and now I had money so didn't really need to do it. I did however agree to take a look and give her a price as a favour. I wasn't sure what the going rate was for tiling a kitchen and I thought I will just have to play it by ear. We arranged that I would call at her house that coming Saturday and we exchanged addresses and phone numbers in case there was any problem in that either of us couldn't keep the appointment.

"You'll be able to meet my kids I have three you know" I got the feeling she expected me to say she never looked old enough but I didn't. I had three children of my own by three different relationships. Apart from Lorna my eldest whose mum Anne I met when we were in care together. I have a daughter Jenna with a girl called Gina, I met Gina through an old friend. I also have a son named James with Paula, an Irish girl I met in a pub would you believe. Unfortunately it is only Lorna that I still had contact with. I know I was not exactly a great advertisement for safe sex but it was a mixture of immaturity and ignorance in that respect. I fell for all of my kid's mothers always assuming that it would be a relationship that would be eternal. There was always something that spoilt it though in the main it was because they looked for greener grass so to speak. I made the decision to walk away on each occasion, I needed loyalty and commitment.

That Saturday was a hot day and I decided to set off early to Carmen's house. I thought I would take my time and walk, in those days I would walk everywhere. I remember stopping at a newsagents for a can of something cold. There was a 40ish year old man in the shop and he was paying me far too much attention. He was with his wife or girlfriend or at that time the term partner was coming into fashion. I started thinking back to a relationship I was once in with a bisexual man and his wife but that man was a lot more straight acting than this guy. They were both on foot, they must have been because when I left the shop with my drink there were no purple cars outside!

I got to Carmen's ten minutes early as it was only about three miles from where I lived. It was an end terraced house and it wasn't until I looked at the piece of paper with her address on again that I realised she had the same door number as me. It was Carmen herself that answered the door to me. "Come through" she said pleasantly. I followed her down a short hallway into the lounge. "This is Brian my husband, Brian this is Tony". I shook his hand with a firm grip. The lounge was quite dimly lit and the walls were stripped and looked to be in the process of being decorated. However, there were still several photos in frames upon one of the walls though. The song coming from the satellite music channel on the telly was 'Going Loco Down in Acapulco' by The Four Tops. Brian invited me through to the kitchen to show me what needed doing. "I want the entire walls tiled floor to ceiling, do you think I have enough tiles?" I looked at the eleven or twelve boxes in the corner of the kitchen between the fridge and the back door. "Should be enough but if not you'll not need to buy many more" I told him. The kitchen was medium sized for that type of house and it had a newly fitted kitchen with a false ceiling. "What colour are the tiles?" I asked him. Carmen shouted through from the lounge, "They are red! It's my favourite colour". Brian frowned and led me back into the lounge.

I told them I could probably do it over the next three Saturdays and gave them a ridiculously cheap quote of around £50. "Can you not do a few hours on a Sunday?" Brian asked. "Afraid not I am busy on Sundays" I was offered and accepted a can of Lager from Brian. I made some conversation about lots of people having red kitchens these days. The song now playing was, 'Real Gone Kid' by Deacon Blue. "I really like this song" I said. With that Brian used the remote control on the arm of his chair to switch the channel to a sports channel. "Don't even know what it's doing on that channel" he said grumpily. My thoughts were at it again a band with blue in their name what could it mean? Brain was a massive guy very stocky with a shaved bald head (this was years before it was popular amongst middle-aged men). Brian must have been ten years older than Carmen. I could see from the trophies on the fire surround that he was or used to be a boxer. I hissed in a jovial way when Brian told me he was a Man United fan. The conversation got around to music and I remember saying I had a catholic taste and laughed when Brian said, "So can't you come after church on Sunday then?" I explained that I liked every kind of music "I particularly like Reggae" I said. "Oh yeah like who?" I was very careful not to mention Bob Marley and said, "John Holt, Gregory Isaacs, Sanchez, Audrey Hall and others". Carmen gave what seemed like a triumphant laugh and said, "Most white people only know Bob Marley!" Brian looked across at her from the armchair where he was sat but said nothing. That seemed to be the end of that topic as he quickly said, "I work the door at different clubs in town". I should have guessed as he had that bouncer look about him. "So where are the kids?" I asked. "At my mothers but they will be here next Saturday" said Carmen. I drained the last of the lager from the can and declined the offer of another realising I had been there for almost twenty minutes. It was agreed I would be back to do the tiling each Saturday from 10am until around 3pm. I stressed that it may only take me two weeks but three to be on the safe side. "I'll see you Monday Carmen bye for now Brian nice meeting you". With that I made my way home.

The following day being Sunday meant it was my day for illegal activity! It had been for the past nine months or so that I did a 5 hour slot on a pirate radio station. For the past six months it was from an 8th floor flat in the block opposite mine. Pirate radio is usually linked to the nightclubs and in particularly the music played in both legal clubs and shebeens and this station was no different. No different that is except for the slot I did as I never had much to do with clubbing being more of a pub person. I very rarely spoke on air so I never mentioned people or places and events or deejays. I did however stick to an acceptable playlist, until recently I would be stoned whilst playing the records. I would play tapes and vinyl LP tracks which were mainly reggae and sometimes I would play a bit of acid house stuff which I borrowed from a neighbour. It was risky because I didn't want to 'frighten the horses' so not that much and not too often. CD's hadn't fully caught on yet although I had made a start at replacing the albums that I had on vinyl. Reggae seemed to be what the masses wanted I say masses but we had no idea of knowing exactly how many people listened in. There was some slight advertising with fliers that were left or given out in clubs or shebeens. I would have loved to play country music, jazz, pop and other stuff I have in my own collection but I just couldn't.

The guys who owned the equipment and ran the station were not exactly model citizens because they were involved in lots of other and more serious illegal activities. Floyd the guy I used to get my cannabis from had had his transmitters confiscated by the DTI on more than one occasion. It usually meant he or whoever was on air would have to escape via the balcony to either the floor below or above (or even further up or down!). It meant getting new equipment and finding a suitable empty flat in another block to set up all over again. Usually there would be a spotter or somebody on lookout but it wasn't always possible as it is a tedious task. The person doing it at the moment only did it because his reward would be getting stoned for free.

It was my mate Jay who introduced me to Floyd and I had known Jay since school. I became involved (only in the radio side of things I hasten to add) because I was able to reinstate the power at the empty flats. I have a good working knowledge of electricity thanks to one particular Youth Training Scheme. The consumer units used by the electricity board were fairly simple to isolate and bypass, therefore allowing me to restore the power supply. Floyd would have readily paid me for this (if not in cash perhaps in weed) but I negotiated some airtime instead. Sundays are not exactly primetime in fact possibly the worse time of all. It was me who suggested and fitted 'door bells' with no sound just a light bulb that would flash. It wasn't pressed from the outside of the door but inside just below the letterbox so you had to put your hand through. Unless you knew it was there you would knock on the door. It was simple but effective and it allowed us to determine whether it was 'friend or foe'. Drugs were never dealt from the flats that were used for broadcasting although drug use in them did happen. We decided for this station not to use a flat that was too high up the block but to lengthen the cable used for the antenna. I think that is why we had managed to evade detection for the past six months. The antenna was laid flat on the roof of the block when no broadcasting took place.

That Sunday I woke at around 5.45 am and it looked as though it was going to be great sunny day. In those days not only did I read newspapers but I had them delivered. As yet my Observer had not hit my front door mat. I tended to read the Guardian because growing up in a 'family group home' I would be sent to the shop to get it. Back then I only ever knew it as the Manchester Guardian. I did try reading the various tabloids but they seemed more about gossip than news, page three girls, celebrities, bingo and a complete waste of money I always refer to them as 'shit sheets'. They have their own agenda and no matter what anybody says they do try to influence the way we think. By the time the newspaper did arrive I had washed, shaved, dressed and eaten my fry-up breakfast. It was a glorious morning outside so I opened the door on my balcony. I turned on the television it was morning worship so I changed the channel and it was Tarzan, I wasn't really watching Tarzan but left it on. Ten minutes later whilst in the kitchen washing the breakfast plate and the frying pan I realised that there was a voice I vaguely recognised on telly. I thought no it couldn't be they wouldn't would they? I went into the lounge and sure enough Tarzan was on, but no Cheetah or Jane the feature had finished. It was Michael Heseltine and I remember laughing and thinking somebody at the BBC had a sense of humour. I was out of cigarettes so went to the local shop which was only 5 minutes away.

When I returned it was Margaret Thatcher who was on the television and I don't even know now what she was talking about but she was wearing a dark colour navy blue I think. I immediately switched the telly off telling her (as if she could hear me) "I did not invite you into my house so get out I don't like you and am disgusted with you!" Then I called her an unctuous cow. In my urgency to get her out of my lounge I had kicked over half a cup of tea onto my new carpet. I looked across over the green area at the rear of my block to the block opposite and I could see the antenna on the roof. I turned the radio on and tuned it away from radio 4 but couldn't pick up my pirate colleagues so they must have left the antenna up from Saturday night.

At half past twelve or so Jay dropped off the key for the broadcasting flat. He didn't stay too long and was obviously under the influence of some street drug or other. Whilst he was at my flat he did tell me that Floyd was concerned and aggrieved that I had found another dealer for getting my weed. "I don't smoke it anymore Jay" I told him. "Yeah right" he said sarcastically. "Is he that desperate for five quid a week?" I asked. "Dunno, but he knows someone else who knows how to do the electrics too". I didn't say anything but I knew that this Sunday was going to be the last time I was going to be broadcasting and I was already thinking of doing it my way. "When are me and you gonna go for a drink then?" I asked. Jay smiled saying, "You know where I go drinking I'll see you in there". Yes I knew where he drank and although the place never had sawdust on the floor it was the type of place where even the arms of the chairs had tattoos. Jay left shortly after smoking the joint which he had assured me was good shit. He had offered to share it with me at least four times. I could see why peer pressure is always put forward as a reason for people getting involved in drug use. I was steadfast though and didn't partake but according to Jay that was because I already had some before he arrived.

I didn't waste any time I started to go through my record collection - LP's, 45's and tapes too. I had just over an hour to compile a list of tracks to fill a five hour slot. After half an hour I had scribbled down about two hours worth of music. I stacked the albums and singles into the order that the tracks were to be played. I was getting really excited imagining that this would be my very own 'Desert Island Discs'. I owned a Sony walkman CD player and had quite a varied selection of CD's. I decided I would sacrifice the headphones and a microphone that I had for the sake of my art. I cut the phones off with a pair of scissors leaving just the length of wire with the small jack plug at one end. I did the same with the mic leaving the wire with a bigger jack plug at that end. I used my teeth to strip away the plastic to reveal the bare wires then I joined the two together making sure none of the wires were touching. I tried it in my own hi-fi plugging the bigger jack plug in and the other end into the phones of the Walkman. I played a CD on the walkman using the auxiliary setting of the hi-fi. I was delighted when the music came through the speakers perfectly. I used some masking tape to insulate the wires then taped it all tidily together.

I arrived on the 8th floor at the broadcasting flat at around 1.30pm carrying a medium sized suitcase and a carrier bag. The bag was full of CD's and in the case I had the walkman, the vinyl and cassettes. I realised that the equipment only had three jack sockets (not counting headphone ones) and that all were taken. If I wanted to I could remove the ones for tape, turntable or microphone at any given time (ie. when they were not in use). I opted to switch between tape and walkman. I was on a mission and everything was going right for me it was exhilarating. On that Sunday afternoon I strung together four and a half hours of eclectic music. I played all sorts of stuff both old and new. Bands like The Smiths, Simply Red, The Housemartins, Beatles, U2, The Blow Monkeys and Deep Purple. I played artists like Brooke Benton, Bryan Ferry, Patti Page, Bowie, Eddie Floyd, Sam Cooke and Ray Charles to name but a few. I played songs like Blue Velvet, Red Red Wine, Mellow Yellow, Pink Cadillac, Green Grass of Home and Pink Floyd's 'Any Colour You Like'. I played Johnny Cash's Orange Blossom Special, Elvis's Blue Suede Shoes, and even Dolly Parton's Coat of Many Colours. I played everything and anything that I had in my collection. It was not all colour related and I was surprised at how many 'colour songs' I did have. I just played what I considered to be great songs, bands or artists. Of course I played some reggae but I also played jazz, blues, country, indie, house and pop. I was having a ball a real adrenaline rush I was totally straight but buzzing out of my tree. I also had a rant about the government and I told a few gags in between the songs. I was so confident it was as if having a conversation or chat with one other person. There was no feedback or interaction but to me that one other person out there was hanging on my every word. I was on top of the world a feeling of being high. High in mood and a feeling of confidence there was nothing I could not accomplish.

I say four and a half hours because at half past six the light bulb above the door flashed several times. It was Jay closely followed into the room by Floyd. "Don't smoke anymore eh?" Jay said in a jokey way. I could tell Floyd was not at all happy but he remained quite calm. "You got some balls Scally what dya think this is the rass clart BBC?" he said. "There's no way the BBC would play all that I have in one show". I could tell from his face I had just pissed him off even more. "I don't fuckin' blame them gimme the fuckin' key". Trying to help me Jay said, "It wasn't all bad, and a lot was coming through loud and strong". As I handed over the key to Floyd I looked at Jay and pointed to the walkman. "CDs, no crackles, hisses or scratches but crystal clear" I said. "Get your shit together I don't want to see you again unless you want weed" said Floyd. I packed away the albums and singles into the suit case and was putting the CDs into their cases when Floyd said, "We are keeping the walkman for the station". He smiled widely showing a back gold tooth. I knew it was pointless to argue and didn't even protest I was just hoping he wasn't going to tell me he wanted my CDs too. As I left the flat I heard Jay consoling Floyd. "If anyone tries to take the piss man just tell them it wasn't our frequency".

In the lift going down I was thinking it could have been much worse and still a feeling of elation I was in the 'Zone!' I had thoughts of all the commercial radio stations offering me contracts. At ground level I walked out into the sunshine and along the path that cut across the green to my block of flats. The case and carrier bag seemed heavier going back although in reality the bag was lighter. It was Floyd who shouted from the balcony above and behind me. "Hey! Tony Blackburn I'll have sputnik on Tuesday". I turned looked up, put down the case and carrier bag (containing all but two of my own CD's) and shouted, "Nah it's okay I gave it up". He shouted "Ya know where I am if ya change ya mind". I shouted back up to him that my jokes were better than Blackburn's and I never heard it but I sense he kissed his teeth.

Back in the bed-sit it wasn't until I was halfway through putting the music away that I noticed an orange stain on my carpet. I felt the area and it was still a bit damp and it was then I remembered spilling the tea earlier. It was ordinary tea a little bit of milk no sugar I couldn't quite believe it. "How on earth has that happened?" I said out loud (talking to oneself is something I think most people who live alone do now and then). It was a terrific colour the orange though and quite unique for a carpet. The original colour of the carpet was a wine coloured burgundy sort of affair. I liked the orange colour so much that I spent the next three hours or so brewing pots of tea. I strategically poured it so as to cover the whole of the carpet. The only areas I left out were out of view like under the bed and behind the telly corner unit. I thought it has to be a dodgy dye used in the manufacture of the carpet but to be on the safe side I will change my brand of tea bags!

I slept with the balcony door open that night and at about 2am I soon realised why I had done so. I squelched from the bed to the bathroom in the dark cursing bloody Margaret Thatcher all the way. Whilst drying my wet orange feet in the bathroom I recalled the time I sent a letter to Thatcher. It was to ask her to spare a thought for Argentinean mothers. I thought all letters to all MPs were responded to but I never heard a thing not even a standard reply. Since that time I have often thought it was a big mistake to write. I am on a list now somewhere and they have me down as a subversive. For the return trip back to bed in order to maintain dry white feet I dived from the doorway onto the end of the single bed. The two legs at the foot of the bed broke and the base dropped at that end with a loud creaking sound as the wood snapped. I remember thinking to myself as I drifted back off to sleep (my head higher than my feet) that the bed breaking was the only thing that had gone wrong for me today.

Chapter Two: It started with a kiss

Despite what people say or sing about Mondays or Monday mornings I was never too bothered or stressed by them. It was looking like it was going to be another warm day. I was stood at the bus stop waiting for my bus to work, I would have liked to have walked but I knew that it would make me late. Just as I was about to chance walking to the next bus stop the bus arrived. As usual once on the bus I made my way upstairs and sat right at the back. A couple of seats in front of me were two youngish lads probably sixteen or seventeen they were talking about some rave or other that never quite happened. This was in the era of the Hacienda and 'Madchester'. I was looking at the traffic, front doors, cars and pedestrians in my now familiar way. I overheard the older of the two boys relate to the other about the various colours and about being very careful. I immediately thought Ah Ha! So I am not the only one who is clueing up on this. I wasn't catching all of what was being said and with hindsight think he may have been talking about various pills or tabs available at raves. They must have thought me totally bonkers though when I think about it now but as I passed them to leave the bus I turned and said, "I am a blue!" lifting the pale blue tie I was wearing. Then as I got to the top of the stairs I turned and said, "And I am not as green as some people think!" I happened to be wearing a blue tie with a white shirt but that's not entirely why I had called myself a blue. The two lads on the bus didn't know it but were influential in me taking a much keener interest from now on in what strangers said. I became convinced something big was happening or going to happen and it may be nationwide but most definitely here in Manchester. I also got the impression that it was all said for my benefit it was contrived and possibly even scripted somehow. I was at the centre of it, but of what though, and why me.

As I walked from the bus stop to work I began to consider the colour thing again. I imagined that somehow years ago somebody had come up with the idea of linking colours to certain allegiances. It is quite true when you think about it with flags, uniforms, logos, and football teams but I was thinking more about the colour keeping a person safe. I needed to find my safe colour and I don't mean something I can get away with at a dinner party! I have been a follower of Manchester City FC for as long as I can remember but if I was blue what of my family? They all support Manchester United FC and I am the only blue they are all reds! I began to think it had nothing to do with football or maybe that's just part of it. I clocked in at work with ten minutes to spare. Carmen had called in sick and the first thing I saw stuck to the monitor at my desk was a yellow coloured post-it note.

'Take care of stock enquiry / part identification today – Dave'.

It involved identifying parts with minimal information at the customer's request meaning no part number or stock code. It usually meant faxing pages from the service manuals of the appliances concerned (exploded diagrams etc). We could then identify/locate the part from stock or order it if not in stock. This was what Carmen usually did as well as the stock control. Liz was doing stock control so it seemed all the more hectic on the phones being two people down. I was dealing with the ordinary calls and as of lunchtime there had been none of Carmen's work for me to deal with.

During lunch whilst the telephones were surprisingly quiet I got into a conversation with Ian about purchasing a home computer for myself. Ian was a bit of a 'gadget person' and a little bit of a show off. He said, "You know I have a 'sharp IQ' and you don't!" I thought for a moment about what he had said and again it was one of those times where I felt this person is telling me something significant here. He was inferring something or giving me a clue! Does he know what's going on and I don't. Is he fully aware or like me feeling his way and trying to suss it all out. Liz and Peter had gone for a pub lunch and Ian asked if I wouldn't mind holding the fort for half an hour on my own as he had to go out on personal business. "No problem". I sat there in the silent office trying to get my head around whatever it is I need to discover or expose. I looked down at the keyboard then the monitor and in the search box on screen I typed 'IQ' and almost immediately it came up with a personal handheld electronic organiser. Phew! So he was telling me I needed some sort of device to find out what the hell it is that is going on or going to happen. I need like a filing system with a better memory than mine but it needs to be smaller than a computer it needs to be portable perhaps. I hadn't made any notes so far it was all in my head. Perhaps he was just using the words as I thought initially does he know what all this is about and I don't because he has a 'sharp IQ'. I liked Ian he had a kind of way about him that suggested he was on top of everything always calm and unstressed. He knew his stuff when it came to electronics too I remember asking him once whether he had Japanese blood in him. Every so often whilst the phones were quiet he would give us all a pop quiz. He'd give us a stock code and we would have to come up with the part number or vica-versa. I would not kid myself that I knew as much as Ian but I would always be top scorer in his quizzes.

I got home that evening and the light on the answering machine was flashing to indicate a message. I picked up the handset and telephoned Vera. "Hiya Mam, what's up?" She said, "Nothing why, what do you mean?" Not many people have my telephone number so I assumed it was Vera who had left a message. "Doesn't matter" I said. I asked about Lorna and invited myself to Sunday Dinner (now being available on Sundays). I had a short conversation finding out what my brothers and sister were up to and I told her I would phone again before Sunday and replaced the receiver. I then pressed play on the answering machine and the message was from Carmen and it took me a few moments to recall giving her my number. "Hi Tony its Carmen, can you telephone me when you get this message it's important but do not phone before eight thirty! Thanks Bye". She had emphasised the 'do not'. I played it again she had a very sexy voice softly spoken with the words spaced out evenly, it was something I hadn't noticed before. I began to think it somewhat emphasised or exaggerated but told myself that lots of people have their own telephone voice. Some even have a voice especially for answering machines but still I found it sort of erotic.

Shopping and cooking for one was something I had gotten used to but sometimes it meant having the same meal the following day. I had purchased a microwave especially for that purpose (reheating). Spaghetti bolognaise actually tasted better the following day I found (the sauce that is). Jay had arrived and was in a bit of a state, put simply he was drugged up. I asked had he eaten and offered to feed him. He was stood shifting from one foot to the other in the kitchen apparently he hadn't eaten in a few days. I asked him to pass me the tennis racket that was stuck in the gap between the fridge and lower cupboard. I could see the needle marks on his arm as he gave me the racket but said nothing.

"Am I tripping or do you have a tennis racket in your kitchen?" he asked. I smiled and used the racket to strain the spaghetti. It wasn't an ideal utensil but I never lost that much into the sink. "Why don't you get a sieve?" I kept meaning to purchase a colander but I never corrected him.

I didn't own a dining table as I usually ate from the plate on my knee or placed the plate next to me on the bed (when it had its legs). His coordination was such that I moved and placed the bedside cabinet in front of my only armchair. The cabinet had looked odd being so high next to the low bed base now. Looking even odder was the contrast in colours of the carpet below compared to everywhere else. He asked why I had taken the legs off the bed and what was with the carpet. I said something about wanting the flat to look like a students gaff. He said, "Mad fucker, you are!" Jay left soon after eating the meal saying something about feeling weird. The purpose of his visit I never got to the bottom of I just assumed it was a social call as he did live in the same block.

I had gotten sidetracked doing some cleaning around the flat before I remembered I must ring Carmen. I fished out her number from the several scraps in my 'don't lose' shoe box and I rang her at ten past nine. It was Carmen who answered almost immediately. "It's Tony what's up?" To start with she said it wasn't anything important just that she wanted to know what had been said at work. I reminded her that she had used the word important in her message. "Well it is but nothing for you to worry about". I told her nothing had been said to me apart from her calling in sick. "Is something wrong?" It was for the next few minutes I just listened as she spoke slowly and softly. She told me that she wasn't sick but that the child minder had let her down and then the flood gates opened so to speak. Speaking more quickly she said it was her husband he had 'gotten to' the child minder. She started telling me that Brian handled all the money and that sometimes he stayed out all night. She told me he cheats on her and never pays the bills and that he doesn't let her have any friends. She said it all in a matter of fact way and still in the husky voice which was new to me. I felt awkward and I told her I was very sorry and asked when she would be back at work. At the risk of sounding mercenary I also enquired whether I was likely to be paid for the tiling. She said that the childminder was phoning her back that evening and if she could not sort it out her sister would mind the youngest as the girls were at school anyway. I asked whether she could speak to a family member about being unhappy at home. She told me her husband had hit her before and if it happened again she was going to leave him. It would mean giving up her job which she loved but her family would support her 100% if they knew she had been hit. She told me that they all lived too far away for her to travel to work. I asked about the tiling money again hoping I could get out of doing it. "I still want you to do the tiling and you will get the money". I told her I would see her at work in the morning I didn't know what else to say and there was an awkward silence for a moment or two. "Why are you telling me all of this?" I asked her. She told me she doesn't know why but thinks I am a genuine person and she can trust me and there is nobody she can really speak to. I felt so sorry for her and thought what is wrong with that man she is absolutely gorgeous.

The next morning not unlike any other male my age I woke with an erection. On the square of burgundy carpet next to the top end of the bed (I hadn't put the cabinet back yet) I could see from the flashing red light I had not erased the message from Carmen on the answering machine. I used my left hand to play it over and over and the other to masturbate.

As usual I was on time for work as was everyone else including Carmen. I decided I was going to let her be the first to start a conversation with me although I did say, "I'm glad you're ok" after she had told Liz that she was fine now. She just smiled at me and what a smile she has. The phones were not as busy as the previous day but Carmen did get several part identification enquires and I think I told her more than once that I didn't receive any yesterday. I thought it odd at lunch time that she was asking the others what they wanted on their sandwiches as I hadn't known Carmen to leave the office during lunch. She openly invited me to go along with her on the sandwich run saying, "I don't buy cigarettes and I know you need them". To which I replied, "Oh dear, does that mean that I have got to actually breathe fresh air then?" It was Liz the chain smoker who found it the funniest her laughter quickly and ironically turned into a cough.

The sandwich shop was about ten or twelve minutes on foot and no sooner were we into minute one when Carmen said, "I know you don't get paid until Thursday but do you have any money you can lend me?" I said, "Course it's only a sandwich". She said, "No I've got to pay the phone bill final demand by this afternoon or it'll be cut off" I heard myself asking how much knowing that I would have enough and had already decided to lend it to her. "£53 should cover it". Without asking when I would get it back we both headed in the direction of the Lloyds Bank where I withdrew £60 from the hole in the wall. I gave it to her and she paid the bill at the same branch and I went in with her. It was whilst she was paying the bill that I felt a sense of disappointment in her and an inevitability that I wouldn't be repaid. Disappointed in myself too for seeming an easy touch and a bit of a mug but at the same time I wanted her to be in my debt. For some reason this was mixed in with my thoughts on why a place so full of money has the biros chained to the counter.

Not much was said returning with the sandwiches but for part of the way it was Billy Ocean's 'Caribbean Queen' that I was humming. I was so grateful that this beautiful, beautiful woman gave me the time of day (even if I was paying for the privilege). I thought about Cleopatra thinking well my name is Anthony! For some reason my thoughts suddenly turned to the song I was thinking about in particularly the word 'queen'.

It was whilst the others and Carmen were eating that I started to think that chess somehow played a part in what it was that was going on. Chess because I couldn't think of anything more tactical or complex involving the colours black and white (are they colours or shades?) Moreover I thought perhaps she may be part of it all and setting me up. Although nobody knew it I had made the first move just like in the game of chess white moves first but who was it who was controlling the game. How could they possibly know of my early morning activities with the phone message? I am being second guessed and somebody is more than one move ahead! I began to think about Kevin Burnett who is the man who taught me how to play chess. Kevin Burnett was a bachelor in his late 40s he wore cravats and did crosswords. I spent a lot of time with him he was very clever and my housemaster at the CHE (Community Home with Education). I lived at the community home from the age of 13 to 16 because the courts placed me into the care of the local authority. There was an air of confidence about Kevin Burnett like somehow he was independently wealthy and worked for nothing at least that's how I thought of him back then. Mr. Burnett (I never called him by his first name to his face) taught me the rules of chess and played several games with me, always winning. Only a few games because two or maybe three weeks into the tuition he became my abuser. Since that time I tended not to play chess, because of the memories it evokes. Puberty was just beginning for me and I was very confused. I was manipulated by a very clever (and devious) man. Confused because it was a father figure scenario and I trusted him and confused because he told me it was love. I felt a sense of shame though and telling nobody ever. He knew how to put the onus onto me and I soon learnt that being good at tossing him off or blowjobs meant being buggered by him less likely.

As I write this I still feel a sense of guilt, shame and somehow that I still feel I need to justify myself.

Suddenly I thought, Oh my God! I know he set me up for the abuse but was it the start of what is happening now? Has it been going on that long and I wasn't aware? In a matter of seconds situations and events throughout my life flashed through my head. "TONY! Are you okay your hands are shaking?" Ian said. "I don't feel too clever, if you can give me five minutes to wash my face" I said looking around the office. "Course you can mate". The others in the office were all looking at me including Carmen who was on the phone. It was the first time Ian had called me mate and it seemed ingenuous enough. It was as if he knew or had realised that for me the penny had dropped and he was wearing a white shirt so he must be an ally! I don't know how I managed to get through the rest of the day without freaking out totally.

That afternoon I did my fair share of answering of the phones although my concentration wasn't good. Account holders would request parts and I was preoccupied with thoughts and suspicions that a third party was listening in on the call. I was becoming more and more suspicious of the people I was interacting with and noting the colours of all the office staff's clothing. Before leaving work I went to see the secretary Janet and booked two days holiday for the following week. I was getting really worried as to whether I was strong enough to get through this and also aware that there wasn't anyone I could confide in.

At home after work I tried to put some things down onto paper but after half an hour or so I realised how little I actually knew and how very complicated it was. I had flow charts, lists, names, songs, key life events and of course colours. I never ate that evening because I had no appetite but on my way home I had bought a cheap bottle of wine and 40 Regal. I remember being in a quandary whether to buy red or white so I edged my bets with rosé. I listened to the radio whilst reading the newspaper and each headline and sub headline was directed at me. The radio was interrupting my reading normally I can get away with it in the background but not today. I switched it off thinking it was purposely trying to distract me from finding the answers in the paper. I found myself reading down the right hand columns of text taking the last word of each line. I don't recall the exact words now but on this occasion it made no sense. I spent some time looking for anagrams too. The Electricity had conked out at one point and I remember putting in several 50 pence pieces. Thanks to the fermented grape I did sleep that evening but only until about 3am. I knew that I had had the most exhilarating and enlightening dream which I had no memory of the instant I tried to recall it. I switched the radio on it was the world service so I started to tune away from it and tuned right into Doris Day singing, 'Que Sera Sera'. I was meant to hear it and it was especially for me! Of all the songs to be played and at that time in the morning it just had to be meant for me personally to hear. It was so profound and it gave me a 'modus operandi' a brand new outlook and philosophy to get through my days from now on, 'Whatever Will be will be'. I had told myself before though that I was going to stop being paranoid and thought by stopping the dope smoking I would be okay but somehow it was as if I was still under the influence of the cannabis at times. I found an elastic band and put it around my left wrist it wasn't tight but wasn't likely to come off unless I took it off. I needed something visual to keep me reminded and to be extra sure on the back of the same hand I put a waterproof plaster from my first aid box. Of course I didn't know I was unwell at the time but I did know I was beginning to get frightened by my own thoughts.

I spent the rest of the week at work with the same thoughts and feelings but now in defiant mood and a lot less anxious. I got several enquiries about my hand and I lied that I had a small gash I also lied about how I had done it (fitting a carpet). As for the elastic band only one person did ask and I just said it was a fashion statement. For some reason though I felt it was as if the elastic band and plaster were both like talisman and would keep me safe.

Carmen and I were becoming good friends as we seemed to be on the same wavelength both being twenty four. The others in the office were in their 30s except Liz the oldest in her late 40s. Carmen had nicknamed me Oscar because of the amount of food I would eat during lunch (Oscar was a character from Sesame Street). According to Liz I must have a tapeworm because I ate like her son and he has one for sure. No matter how much I ate (usually a lot) I was and remained very slim in those days.

We were having terrific weather that summer and the Saturday morning that I walked to Carmen's house must have been one of the hottest days of the year. I became really self conscious about the colours of the clothing that I wore and on that particular day I had changed my clothes at least three times. I decided eventually to wear all white except for the trainers. They were clothes I had had for a while and clothing ideal for the weather but probably too good for working in. Carmen opened the door to me wearing white shorts and a white top. "Snap!" I said and she laughed as I stepped over the doorway. "I thought you said your kids would be around" I said looking at the photographs of the three of them on the wall. "Oh they are with my mum". I walked into the kitchen telling her I'd just get on with it. I worked for about 40 minutes before being offered a drink I had asked for tea but she only ever drank chocolate. I settled for orange juice which I downed in one. It was not working weather more like beer garden weather I thought. After about another hour or so I had done half of the longest wall. I went into the lounge where Carmen was sat watching telly and I told her I was just popping out for a smoke. I made my way down the hall and through the front door out onto the street leaving the door ajar. As I smoked my cigarette I got an overwhelming feeling of being watched and I can't explain it other than to say it was how I felt. About an hour later I had almost finished the biggest wall and I remember so vividly and as if it happened just yesterday. I was squatting down in order to put in the last few bottom tiles when she tapped me on the shoulder. I stood and turned and before I knew it she was kissing me on the mouth. This hadn't happened to me before and all that went through my mind was how gorgeous she was and how things like this you only read in cheap men's magazines. I thought of the time two years previously that I got involved in a ménage à trois but I wasn't seduced more a case of when the work was finished the husband offered to pay me to go with his wife. I could almost hear my own heart pounding and somehow we ended up in the lounge and it was from there that I heard a definite noise from the room above! I immediately pulled away from the kissing and she whispered, "Don't worry he won't get up". I removed her hand from my shorts and said "This is not a good idea". It had only been two or three minutes since that first kiss with both of us still standing. "I better go and change" she said quietly and left the room. She was wearing the same top but had jeans on when she came back down stairs. I pointed to what was obviously still an erection beneath my shorts and said, "Listen I have to go". Before leaving I finished off the last few tiles on the kitchen wall thinking Brian would think it odd if it was left as it was. I told her I was not in work now until Wednesday but that she needed to telephone me. I asked her to get me a taxi because there was no way I could walk home the way I was. "I will but I want you to know I want to be with you". Very quietly almost whispering I said, "I don't want to discuss anything now just phone the cab". I was having visions of him coming down stairs whilst I was still in the state of arousal. Nothing else was said or done until the taxi arrived when I adjusted myself as best I could as I stood from the chair. "See what you have done to me" I said pointing at Mr. Happy again. She smiled and we said bye.

The taxi was a black cab and apart from asking my destination there wasn't any conversation until we arrived. The driver happened to be female and attractive too and I wondered whether she might have known I had a hard-on. The more I thought about that the harder it felt. She wouldn't let me leave the cab unless I left my wristwatch as insurance and the meter was left running whilst I went up to the flat. I decided to forfeit the cheap watch for the already £6 fare mainly because I really needed to sort myself out. Which is exactly what I did on and off for the next few hours replaying the events of the day like a cheap flick in my mind.

It was whilst I was in the bath at about 11pm that I started to really consider what had happened without it being a huge turn on. I was trying to think as rationally as I could and asking myself why I hadn't realised he was upstairs sleeping. He had already told me last week that he worked in night clubs. Perhaps it was more a case of me wanting it to be that we were alone in the house. There was no point in me pretending that I did not fancy her like mad but she was married. I began to wonder whether the whole thing was a case of her looking for an excuse to leave him. It was whilst I was considering why he may have hit her previously that my telephone started to ring. I stood up in the bath and was about to climb out when I had second thoughts and sat back down. It stopped ringing out and I could hear myself from the other room then the longish beep. It was Vera asking me to let her know whether I was definitely coming for dinner tomorrow. I whacked a bit more hot water in using my toe to turn the tap.

It was later whilst cleaning the bath that the telephone rang out again and again I let the machine take the call. This time it was Carmen and she was asking me to call her back but before 2am stressing the word before. I was aware that nightclubs close at around two in the morning so guessed Brian must be working. The plaster from the back of my hand lay at the bottom of the now empty bath. I was tempted to return the call straightaway but I needed to think about what I might say and whether an affair with her was wise. As for the plaster I wondered just which person it was whose skin was used as a guide for the colour it certainly wasn't me. I had never even considered it before but wondered whether there were flesh coloured plasters for Black people, Chinese and Asian people. It was getting a bit late and I was feeling quite hungry so I made some cheese sandwiches on brown bread and a cup of tea. It was the first thing I had eaten since breakfast and only my third brew of the day. I was enjoying the mandatory cigarette afterwards when the phone started to ring again. I answered it on the third ring (something I had picked up from work) "hello" I said, my heart beginning to race. "It's me Carmen I left you a message earlier" she said softly. "Yes, sorry I was in the bath, then I couldn't find your number" I lied. There was an awkward silence for a few seconds. "How come you aren't in work till Wednesday then?" she asked. I told her I had booked Monday and Tuesday off. "Listen, are we going to discuss what happened today?" I asked. "You know what happened". I told her to hang on a second and I crossed the room and put the cigarette out in the ashtray next to my armchair. "Yes I know what happened but what does it mean?" I asked. "I like you a lot" she responded. "It's mutual but you are married and what's more he is violent". I just knew that however tempting a love affair with this beautiful woman was I mustn't even consider it. I wasn't entirely sure whether it was morality on my part, fear of being found out or what. For the next fifteen minutes or so I said very little whilst Carmen told me how desperately unhappy she was. Apart from the violence her husband wouldn't let her go anywhere and she had no real friends. He never did his share when it came to the children and would have her minding his nieces and nephews as well as their own children. He wouldn't allow her to have driving lessons and if she needed money she had to beg for it. By the time she had finished I knew that she had many valid reasons for being unhappy. I asked her why Brian had hit her. "I fell getting off a bus and hurt my wrist so I went to the hospital to get it checked out" she said. "So what's so bad about that?" I asked. "He didn't believe me so lashed out" she replied. "You said today that you wanted to be with me" I said. "Yes yesterday I did". I looked at the clock on my wall and it was after midnight. "Did you mean you want to have an affair because I am not entirely sure I can do that" I said. Before she could respond I asked her why she didn't just leave him. She said, "It's just not the right time but I don't see a future with him that's for sure". I then said, "Well you and I are now good friends and that can continue and I can be here for you as a friend". Throughout the whole of the conversation I wanted to just blurt out that I was crazy about her but I never. I did however say that perhaps down the line the two of us may have a future together. Then getting off the subject I asked the names of her kids and she told me they were Chloe, Amanda and Jerome. We joked about colleagues at work and I asked whether there was any particular reason red was her favourite colour, "It just is" is all she said. We chatted more about colleagues at work and music, by the time I had replaced the receiver we had been talking for over an hour. I really did find her easy to talk to and began to think that she was the one true person I could trust.

It was after one in the morning and too late to return the call from Vera so I decided that I would do it before I leave the flat later. Even though I hadn't stopped all day, tiled an entire wall and had umpteen wanks I was still wide awake. As well as my record and CD collection I had quite an assortment of books in the flat. They were housed in two smallish book cases and a wall mounted shelf and some were just lined up on the windowsills. They were mostly classics but with some biographies and the odd paperback bestseller. I found a copy of Tess of the d'Urbervilles in amongst them and I must have started to read it again previously as the page was marked with a torn slip of paper. The slip of paper turned out to be part of an ad from some loan company or other. Again it was one of those moments that seemed part of the plan, of all the books I chose that one it was as if I had left myself a clue earlier with the advert. Not just an advert but this was a colour coded advertisement. The phone number and company name must have been just above where it was torn as they were missing -

Don't be put off or worry

about your financial situation,

we are here to help keep

you out of the red and in the black.

Almost immediately the first and last word on each line jumped out at me - 'Don't worry about situation we keep you black!' Who the heck are we I thought and what does keep me black mean? Then I read it in its entirety again and read the small print stating 'your home is at risk if the loan payments are not kept up'. I looked at the numbers on the pages it separated in the book and they never meant anything to me. So I thought about the storyline of the book and dismissed the idea that I was related to some luminary or other and that Tess represented my daughter Lorna. I thought about another Hardy novel, 'Far From the Madding Crowd' and I seemed to recall being told that the title came from a gravestone! I thought about Carmen and the game of chess but chess is a war game, surely I am not caught up in a war! I wondered about the colours black and white and then red and decided this must be more subtle than chess, cards perhaps. She was the queen of hearts that would make her red and after all it was her favourite colour. I wondered who the Aces were and I guessed Brian may be the king being married to the queen. I thought perhaps he would be the king of clubs with him being a bouncer around the clubs of Manchester. But that made him a black king and her red queen. Then I thought of song titles and lyrics like the 'Ace of Spades' by Motorhead and 'from a Jack to a King' by Jim Reeves. There was also that deck of cards song where the soldier had no Bible and other songs like 'Diamonds Are a Girl's Best Friend'. Cards are a game of chance though surely this isn't about fluke or even probability or is it. I asked my self plenty of questions but came up with nothing that gave a clearer idea and I wished I knew the phone number of the company. Thinking more about how Carmen or Brian fitted into it all I decided that tonight was the night I was going to get it all straight in my head. Phrases like the cards are stacked against me and being dealt a bum hand ran through my mind. The only things I could think of involving both colours red and black apart from cards was roulette, a ladybird, a poppy or a butterfly. Perhaps that one piece of paper said it all then maybe it was all to do with money. I just wasn't getting a clearer picture but the butterfly linked me into thinking back to when I was a teenager I worked weekends as DJ (I was paid in beer). It was at a pub called the 'Red Admiral' so my thoughts jumped to that time in my life looking for clues.

I thought about many more things, people, places and songs for the next few hours. Here, I am just trying to give a small example of how my thoughts were going and making links from one thing to another.

It was the telephone that woke me later that morning I answered it without opening my eyes and It was Vera, "Are you still coming for dinner son?" she asked. "Yes, not sure what time though but don't wait for me you eat yours and I will have mine once I arrive". I told her I will phone in a while when I was fully awake. I opened my eyes as I replaced the receiver and looked around at the total mess the room was in. There were books, CDs and LP's strewn across the floor and Post-it notes of all colours were marking different passages and pages on the open books. There were more on album covers, CD cases and on the furniture too. There was a note on the mirror which was off the wall leaning against the chair (the note reading - 'man in the mirror'). Of course the album nearest to it was Michael Jackson's 'Off the Wall' (oddly though the song 'man in the mirror' wasn't on that album). The telly had masking tape stuck to the screen from corner to corner diagonally. The ashtray was almost overflowing with cigarette butts and there were at least five used tea cups on the windowsill.

Just in case you are wondering, I hadn't had drunken monkeys in my lounge it was me!

I recalled the previous hours and the mission that I had been on throughout the night. I must have only had an hours sleep in the past 24 but I had so much energy and at the time I felt like I was Einstein in a lab. Apart from my hair style that morning I had probably been more like some crackpot professor than Einstein though. It all made so much sense to me at the time linking things and remembering conversations, I was so sure I was going to solve everything. With each new thought I had it linked to something else and the closer I was getting to my Eureka moment. There was a yellow post-it note stuck to the wall clock which said 'rock around'. I had put it there because I had remembered earlier that the landlord of the Red Admiral insisted that 'Rock Around the Clock' was played each weekend. This clutter and mess went totally against my usual orderly and tidy environment. I lit my first and last cigarette (first since waking and last in the packet) and put the kettle on. I put all of the post-it notes into the shoebox containing Carmen's phone number and a half filled notepad from a previous long night. Then I spotted the elastic band thinking some reminder you turned out to be but I kept it on thinking it would still keep me protected. The phone rang again and I let the machine take the call. It was Carmen asking if I would skip the tiling this Saturday as she is out buying beds for the kids. I thought that's nice you still owe me £60 lady!

I arrived at my Mam's house at about 1.30pm as well as Lorna and Vera my younger brother Peter was there. I hadn't seen Pete for sometime because he had been in London working in a hotel with my older half brother Thomas. There were five of us kids in the family my two older half brothers George and Thomas, Me and Pete and our younger sister Karla. Pete and I had a closer relationship with each other as I suppose George and Thomas do with each other. My sister wasn't brought up by Vera but by her Mam our Nana. We never saw Karla that often whilst growing up as my Nana lived in Salford and we only ever went for Sunday dinner there very occasionally.

Pete lived with a girl called Beth and they had a son together called Adam. "Alright our kid how you doing?" he said as I entered the living room. "I am okay, you?" I responded. "Not three bad, I am working with Beth's Dad now fitting carpets". I asked him whether the pay was any good. "Not great but am gonna learn to drive and work for myself" he said confidently. Lorna was playing with some dolls and stuff on the floor and as usual the telly was on in the corner of the room. I remember commenting to Vera that there was no way I would invite Jim Davidson into my lounge pointing to the telly. Pete and I had a certain sense of humour that we probably inherited from our Dad. When we were together we would bounce one-liners off each other and tell jokes and try to be clever with it.

Vera and Lorna had already eaten and after Pete and I had finished what is always a great Sunday dinner we went back through to the lounge and lit our fags. Pete looked at me and then Vera and said with a smirk, "Thanks Mam that was nice but could've done with another slice of gravy". My Mam is one of those old fashioned women who has cooked a Sunday dinner every Sunday for the past 40 years or so. The standing joke in the family is to rib her about her cooking, even though I personally haven't tasted better. I asked Pete if he remembered us throwing Yorkshire puddings off the balcony at our old house. He was already laughing before I had commented on how high they had bounced, they never did bounce but I always said that they had. "We were the only kids in Manchester that wanted to go to bed with no supper!" he chuckled. I was getting a bit tired so thinking about making my way home but not until I had had another cup of tea. Whilst Vera was brewing the tea Pete started to talk about our Dad (it's not unusual even now for us to reminisce about him). "Remember when Diver (our Jack Russell) shit behind the telly?" he asked. "You mean the morning after the Charles Bronson film 'Valdez's Horses'?" I said laughing. There was an inordinate amount of crap for such a small dog that my Dad suggested it may have been one of the Horses the night before. We called him Diver because that's what he did, hurled himself onto furniture both front paws together as if diving. "What about the time mi Dad was on the phone to the gas board" I said. He had gotten into a row about an unpaid gas bill and ended the call saying, "I put all of the bills into a hat and if you get pulled out you'll get paid, and

anymore threats you won't be going into the hat!" I
distinctly remember him winking to me as he said it. We
chatted and joked for ages about different things and I
decided to stay the night but don't remember falling to
sleep.

I could hear the birds twittering I was on the couch in
Vera's front room. Sat in the armchair was Andy (my
Mam's boyfriend) he was drinking tea and smoking one
of his roll up cigarettes. Andy said, "have you got work
today it's half six?" I told him I had a couple of days off
and asked what time I had fallen asleep. He said he
didn't know exactly but that Vera had covered me with a
blanket after Pete had left sometime last night. "Our Pete
is having trouble with that Beth she has been attacking
him and bit his arm last week" Andy said. You would
have thought he was talking about a dog unless you
knew Beth was his girlfriend. "Is there any tea in the
pot?" I asked. Andy and my Mam had been together for
years and he and I didn't always get on but he's down to
earth and a decent man.

I took Lorna to school that morning and even though
only 9am it was fairly warm outside. Back at Vera's the
three of us drank tea and were doing the crossword
whilst we waited for the pubs to open. The crossword
was in one of the shit sheets because unlike me Andy
reads the tabloids. As he was giving me the clues I
started to wonder which paper it was and became aware
that it was the Mirror. I took a quick look at it once the
crossword was done and I read a little bit about Iraq
invading Kuwait. I began to recall the song and the post-
it note from the early hours of Sunday morning 'man in
the mirror'. I thought whilst reading, that if you look in a
mirror you see yourself but in reverse. So I deduced that
everything I read was there for me but the opposite of
what was being said. One particular sub headline

contained the words 'lost' and 'alive'. I interpreted this as 'Found Dead!' I told Andy and Vera that if anything happens to me it would not be an accident and Vera told me to stop being daft! I never went into any of the details of the way I was thinking but did say I just had a feeling about it. Vera, me and Andy spent the rest of that day in the several local pubs. I told them both it may be the last ever drink I had with them and to take care of Lorna. I could see that I was upsetting Vera so never mentioned anything further. We drank, played pool, and were playing the fruit machine and winning. I had had my quota as Vera left to collect Lorna so said my goodbyes and made my way home.

I was thinking back to my childhood and my parents those few days that I was off work. I recall thinking about the time Vera had to get stitches above her eye and another time he had tried to lift her up so as to throw her from the second floor flat window. I recalled the time he had given her 'a good hiding' for me cutting my own curls off and how I felt responsible. Then there was the time I woke to see him pull back the corner of the carpet in my room to get the family allowance payment book and me hearing Vera crying downstairs. I thought about all the other times there must have been where I hadn't witnessed my Dad battering my Mam. I recalled times we had to hide and pretend we weren't in because we had no money. The loan shark banging on the door who was known only as 'the club man' and Vera trying to make out that it was just a game we were playing. Somehow because he is now dead both Vera and Pete have head-in-the-clouds view of my Dad and never refer to the abysmal side of his nature. When I have tried to bring up about those times it usually ends up in an argument as if somehow I didn't love him. The truth is I still love and miss him dearly he was my Dad. My Dad was one of the funniest and most intelligent people I have ever known and he was scared of nobody.

When Vera did eventually leave him she had taken us with her to our Nana's. George and Thomas were with their real Dad and had been for quite a while before she left. My Dad turned up at my Nana's half pissed. Our uncle Pat was there and asked us both what no child should ever be asked. "Who do you want to live with your Mam or Dad?" After about twenty minutes of being told we couldn't have them both and a lot of crying we opted for the fun option. There was no question of Karla coming with us as my Nana ensured it was non-negotiable and that she would stay with her and our Granddad who had brought her up, up until then.

From my Nana's house we went directly to the train station and spent the weekend in Blackpool. On the way to the hotel I shit myself for the first and last time since being out of nappies. Nobody knew (except maybe Bob the hotelier) I hid my underpants under the bed at the hotel. When my Dad came up from the bar downstairs he was complaining that the room stunk and tried opening the sash type window. He pushed it up and it came down on his finger and there was a lot of blood and quite a deep cut and Pete and I were crying. The window was definitely faulty in that it had no weights that kept the window in the open position. The hotelier took care of the wound and my Dad being my Dad was on free brandy and no room charge until we left on Sunday. I felt responsible for that and I mean the injury not the silver lining. But I often wonder what Bob thought finding the shitty underpants because my Dad kept insisting that he had definite problems with his drains. I also wonder if he ever relates the story of his guests the Scally's from Manchester in a way that has us down as rogues or freeloaders. This was years before the term 'scallies' or being a 'scally' had ever left Merseyside and became part of the vocabulary of the rest of the country. In Liverpool however the term or name is tinged with a certain degree of admiration 'lovable rogue'. Different parts of the country use the term in differing ways though as for in Blackpool or wherever Bob may live now I am unsure. I remember at the breakfast table my dad asking us if we were sure we had had enough to eat between mouthfuls of what was his second breakfast. After breakfast as we were heading out to the pier he reminded Bob that we may require sandwich's upon our return.

Despite my dads drinking we had a good weekend doing the usual things. We would be in bed whilst it was still light outside with Dad downstairs in the bar hammering Bobs brandy. I would be wide awake thinking about my Mam mainly and wishing I had opted to stay with her. Just how he managed to last the next three months or so without the social services getting involved I just don't know. I found out many years later that my Dad had gotten sole custody of us because he had threatened my Mam with violence if she attempted to turn up for the hearing. The incredible thing about my Dad was that he had only ever hit me once in my whole life and that was for accidentally setting a den on fire with a candle. The den being a double bed base folded into tent position in my bedroom! I am sure it was Pete who had done it (accidentally) but because I was older it was me who had the reddest arse in Manchester that night.

It was fun living with him we would have late night meals cooked on an electric 'baby belling' cooker. The gas had been disconnected and so had the electricity but he had learnt to bypass the meter just as I had done all these years later. Our tea was sometimes from the chippy and we had the telly on till late. There would be random people he'd met at the pub asleep on our couch some mornings. Biscuits, crisps, coke and loud music were the norm and there was often a party atmosphere. We asked him every day about our Mam and he would say, "She has run off with a Blackman!" I remember him buying a door streamer it had long strips of different coloured vinyl to keep the flies out in summer. I don't recall it ever hanging at the front door or any other but what he did do was remove all the plastic strips that were yellow. I would see them blowing outside in the wind as he had trapped them in the closed windows. They were also tied to the balcony posts outside at the front of the flat. Apart from Johnny Cash songs the most played record was 'Tie a Yellow Ribbon Round the Old Oak Tree' which was a favourite of my Mam's. I got to know the words and the basis of the song and would pray that she would 'stay on the bus' with the Blackman where she was safe. I would watch the buses sometimes trying to maybe catch sight of her. There were other things that happened whilst living with my Dad that weren't so much fun. We encountered bullying and ridicule at school and we were called tramps by the other kids. It was apparently common knowledge that we wet the bed and we were told that we stunk. One week we were painted head to foot every morning before school at the local clinic. We were the 'Scally's with scabies' and it was a different smell for them all that week. There was one fur coat (fake) that I would sleep with that never got wet, it was my part of my Mam and my most valued possession in the flat. It must have been about eight weeks or so after Vera left that we moved into the living quarters above the local pub where my Dad was a barman. He was being prosecuted for stealing electricity so we moved out. We were lodgers at the pub if children can be lodgers but if anybody asked us it was our Dad's pub and he was rich. We weren't there for too long and not surprising really with wonderful crisp cotton sheets and warm duvets and us pissing the bed every night. I still missed my Mam and I missed that fur coat. To start with the landlady whose name I don't remember would bring us hot Vimto and was very kind to us. Then as the days went on we became more resented and do I really have to tell you the Vimto stopped coming. The landlord was more like my Dad, a big drinker and easygoing, his name was Norman. I recall he had unfeasible eyebrows that would put Dennis Healey's to shame. One afternoon my Dad didn't turn up to collect us from school and nor had he arranged for anyone else to. We were taken into care and it was all agreed whilst we were in our lessons that day. I should have known that morning but you don't when you're a kid. "Bye Uncle Norman see ya tonight thanks for the crisps". He must have thought poor bastards and maybe wished he had made the effort to give us crisps to eat every morning. Pete and I spent the next year and a half in Care, at first in children's homes then into a family group home. It was voluntary care so not a care order imposed by the courts.

When we first got to the family group home the two house-parents (known as Auntie and Uncle) were fine with us. It wasn't too long though before Auntie started smacking us each morning for the bed wetting. I am not talking slight smacking but very hard on our bare arses, at first with her hand then almost always with a belt. Thankfully those two house-parents soon left and the next Auntie and Uncle never hit us. The bedwetting was stressing them out but on the whole it was a nice place to live. We attended a local school and were actually enjoying school. Uncle tried to teach me at that time how to play chess and although he taught me how some of the pieces moved I never quite got the hang of it. Uncle had his own darkroom and was a keen amateur photographer. As Uncle had a regular job we saw more of Auntie. They were both kind to me and Pete and to the other children in the home. We went on holidays with them and got involved in gardening, the photography and other hobbies. I remember us making our own outfits for a school fancy dress party I was a clown and Pete was a pirate. We still missed our Mam and Dad though but in my case I missed my Mam more. They would visit us every so often and only once did they visit us together. I remember Pete getting excited that they would get back together and get us out of care. I prayed to myself that it wouldn't happen as I didn't want Vera to be hit again. He did take us out of care eventually and we lived with him and his new girlfriend for a short time. I remember that every so often he would get me to sign a post office savings book and for a few moments I actually held the cash. Once there was no money left in the account that Auntie and Uncle had set up for us we were sent to live with Vera and her new boyfriend Andy. Everything was okay until the end of my second year of high school when I got into trouble over truancy and some petty crime. That is when the courts sent me to the community home. This was a care order and there was nothing I could do about it and nobody could come along and get me out. I had to stay at the home until my 16th birthday I was around 13 years old at the time.

It was also during that time off from work that I had cancelled my newspaper subscription. It was becoming harder to concentrate on reading anything these days without 'reading something in to it'. As I have said I also have a bit of a problem with advertising and brand names. The problem with advertising was not just the ads on the radio, telly and newspapers but also the subliminal ones too. Okay so you buy your groceries at 'Kwik Save' and you carry it home in a carrier bag you have paid for. All the way home you are advertising and endorsing that shop and you are paying them for the privilege. I started turning bags like this inside out. Then there were other ads where I was 'told' - "Phone this number now!" or "Don't delay Phone Today!" I would say to myself, 'No! I won't and who's going to make me?' I did wonder all the same whether by phoning just one number I would get to the bottom of everything. Yes that's it it's not all complicated it's just me that must be thick the answers must be there.

Chapter Three: Colour me sad

That First Wednesday back at work in the office I was left holding the fort at lunchtime. I telephoned what used to be 192 (Directory enquiries) and enquired about the telephone number of Jacobs & Co. I was given their head office number which I dialled and it was answered by an extremely cheery lady with a southern accent. "Hello it's about your advert" I said. "Yes sir, how can I help?" she enquired. "I want to join your club!" She giggled and said, "Club sir?" By this time Ian was back in the office so I scribbled 'Jacobs Biscuits' on a scrap of paper and pushed it across the desk for him to read. "Yes, I like a lot of chocolate on my biscuit can I join your club?" I was told, "There is no club Sir it's a biscuit". I told her I could send a cheque for the membership if need be and that would also prove I was Anthony Scally from Manchester! By now Ian was finding it hard to control the volume of his laughter and it was then I realised that Ian was totally in the dark about all that was going on. She went from cheery to snotty and must have heard him laughing because she asked was I serious stating, "It's a biscuit!" I was tempted to sing what the advert stated but just asked, "How can you join a Biscuit then?" She remained silent and I thought Ah Ha! I really am onto something here. "It doesn't make sense!" I said emphatically. Then there was a click… she had hung up on me! Ian still laughing said, "I can't believe you have just made that call and how did you keep a straight face?"

I let him think it was all a joke I had to as I couldn't tell him about my daughter being 'brainwashed' by the advert. I couldn't tell him about 'the king of clubs' and orange is one of the flavours of club biscuits or of my once red but now orange carpet. I didn't tell him of orange being the colour of cream cracker packaging and Dave referring to me as 'crackers'. I definitely wasn't likely to tell him of hiding from the 'club man' and it all being a game. I couldn't tell anyone! I was trying to get through this in one piece like Morse trying to solve a case but unlike Morse I had no Lewis. If there was a Lewis out there for me it definitely wasn't Ian.

As I didn't have to do the tiling that Saturday I did all of my household cleaning whilst listening to the radio. The weather was changing according to the forecast. It had been a great summer but inevitably now that we were into August it was becoming a bit milder. There was a knock at my front door, I opened it and it was Carmen so I invited her in. She was wearing a yellow rah rah type skirt, sandals and a white blouse. "This is a surprise" I said. "I brought your money, thanks for lending it to me". She handed me the three twenty pound notes. She said that Brian was away in London for the weekend. She then told me that he had used the kid's bed money to buy a car and her tone suggested that she wasn't at all happy about that. I was trying hard to keep my eyes off her lovely legs as she sat in the armchair. "Fancy us having the same door number" she said. I just nodded and smiled, all the while wondering what colour her knickers were!

On Sunday morning I woke with her next to me and they were pink and on the floor next to the bed. I moved in the bed and put my arm around her. I realised she was awake so we did what we had been doing throughout the night only that morning it felt even better. I know I had said I wouldn't get involved sexually but an Oscar Wilde quote springs to mind 'I can resist anything but temptation'. Later that afternoon just as she was leaving she told me she was going to leave Brian. I asked if she was sure and what about work, she told me that she had had enough and would find another job once she had found somewhere to live. She mentioned the car he had bought again referring to it as a 'hearse'. I asked what she meant and she said it was a really long car like a hearse. "Is it black?" I asked. "No it is brown". After she had left the flat I really began to feel a bit panicky this could get very dangerous for me and for her. Shit I really need to sort out the code thing before I get into a relationship.

I somehow managed to get through Monday at work without just walking out and coming home I really didn't want to be there. I kept looking at my left wrist and the rubber band upon it thinking whatever will be will be. I tried to look as indifferent as I could do each time somebody mentioned Carmen's name. "She hasn't even bothered to phone in" Ian said. It wasn't until Tuesday that we were informed that she had left the firm and had written a letter. I already knew she had written the letter on that Sunday evening because she had telephoned me. "He has hit me again!" she said. She was phoning from her mothers where she was staying with the kids. "Punched me three times in the head" she told me. I winced as she was telling me and all I could think to say was "Bastard!" She had an appointment with the town hall domestic violence unit and hopefully she would get re-housed soon. We chatted for about forty minutes or so and I told her I would support her in any way she wanted me to. She gave me her Mum's phone number and said I could phone her anytime I liked.

Winter was drawing in it was getting colder by the time Carmen and the children were placed into a safe unit near the Manchester Royal Infirmary. I would visit them some evenings after work and although it was against the rules sometimes I would stay overnight. I met Carmen's brother her three sisters and her mother. I had gotten to know the children a little better they were all still quite young. I knew from my own experience how upsetting parents separating can be. The only good thing was that Brian hadn't hit Carmen whilst they were around. I had had threats from Brian on the phone and Carmen said he must have gotten the phone number from an itemised bill. "You will not reach your 26th Birthday" he told me in a flat even tone. My birthday was in October about three weeks away but it was going to be my 25th. I thought it odd at the time for him to give himself so much time to do whatever he was going to do. I suppose it was a case of 'I'll kill you but its very short notice'. A murder threat was all I needed though especially the way my mind was working. It was as though now I had two problems to contend with.

I was told by Jay that Floyd had been shot dead in London and I realised it was the weekend that Brian was in London. I told myself it's a big place besides boxers don't use guns they have a scrap like men. I wondered also why Brian may want to shoot Floyd unless they were rival criminals. Before leaving the flat Jay helped himself to the money in my wallet whilst I was out of the room. I began to become very suspicious of everyone, strangers and sometimes even people that I knew. I was never that gregarious and preferred my own company anyway so the people I knew were mainly work colleagues or neighbours. Although I got on with my neighbours I purposely wouldn't go into their flats or invite them into mine. It was a conscious decision on my part I don't see myself as a loner but others would see me as that I guess. I had a loose association with Jay through weed smoking sessions and we were good mates but I had stopped smoking weed now. He had moved on to harder drugs and I didn't anticipate seeing him again after the theft of the forty quid. I got my telephone number changed but that didn't stop the overwhelming feelings of being watched or followed. It just didn't feel right at my flat anymore. Carmen had told me more about her life with Brian. She told me of the police searching the house for guns one morning that she was getting the kids ready for school. The time she had found out that he had 'staged' a burglary at their house one Christmas. The gun thing scared me a little but robbing your own house at Christmas I could not get my head around.

Signs and their colours had started to take on even more relevance in that I thought they were specifically there for me 'Please do not smoke', 'Keep Britain tidy' and others. Not just instructions directly aimed at me but potential clues. I had stopped smoking on the buses and had become one of those people with pockets full of sweet wrappers and receipts. I would even look for clues amongst the contents of my own pockets as I emptied them every few days. I avoided the telly, radio and newspapers because it became impossible for me to read, hear or see anything without it taking on significance. I would read backwards, forwards, sideways and analyse every possible meaning of what was written or said. I didn't avoid these things because I didn't want to know what it was all about, I avoided them because there was just too much to take in. The song title, 'Born to Lose', and film title, 'Live and Let Die' I recall reading in the same paragraph in a magazine at the dentist's. The check-up was going to have to wait I thought as I left the surgery like a bat out of hell. Other people's remarks or conversations (not always with me) I would take on board too. For me there had become no such thing as coincidence. One time Carmen commented that 'everything happens for a reason'. Although I trusted Carmen I didn't want to frighten her by trying to explain that I was caught up in the middle of something and for the same reason I hadn't mentioned anything of it to members of my own family either. This was about me I didn't really want to drag anyone else into it. It may sound quite self-interested but I believed and still believe I have a duty to protect my children and without me they are vulnerable or at risk. I also had thoughts that perhaps my Dad had crossed somebody and so from the day I was born because I was his eldest I was a 'target'. Once he had died it passed on to me, there were thoughts of will it end or is it that I need to die to end it! I really had to sort out whatever it was to protect my own children in case it passed onto them if I did die. I decided that if I was going to die I was not going to go without a fight. I was convinced I could work it all out before it got to that though. If it was a game of chess I was reacting to moves and somehow being second guessed or continually on the back foot (not really the way to win a game). Everything was open to scrutiny by me and I mean everything! Everything was said or done for my benefit it was as if other people wanted to 'control' or 'manipulate' the way I was thinking they were trying to steer me in a certain direction. It was like a person would say something but they were acting on behalf of somebody else and that somebody else was using them. Going through them to tell me things or steer my thinking, saying things by proxy if you like. I thought about Thatcher and her advisors and if we got a new government would they be the same advisors. I started to note the brands of cigarettes that people smoked and realised that for some reason a lot had upper-class names or were even to do with the monarchy. Just something posh about them names like Berkley, Sovereign, Dorchester, Consulate, Embassy, Regal and lots of others. There were coats of arms or crests on some of the packets too. My interest was not just in cigarette packets but lots of inanimate objects. It didn't matter if it was a plastic comb, a key ring, a toy car or an apple in a fruit bowl. The position or colour or both things combined, it all held clues. It was symbolism nothing was as it seemed it was all representing or alluding to something else. I believe there is a secret language that we all recognise but few are fluent in and it's the language of symbols. Symbols surround us in numerous forms and form an inextricable part of our daily lives, yet unlike our spoken languages schooling in symbolism is left to the individual initiative. The problem for me was that everything and I mean everything began to symbolise something, something that was pertinent to my own life and situation. It was also part packaging or branding of everyday things, companies, advertising, you name it from board games to hosepipes. Logos and the colours of logos and the fonts it was all scrutinised by me. Most people scrutinise wage slips, and show an interest in the football team they follow and be interested in things that concerned them personally. I was no different but it was the way I would assimilate the information that was very different and the trouble was everything seemed to concern me personally. Some days I would feel like James Bond on a mission when I say feel like Bond I mean quite invincible and not in anyway afraid. I had a kind of secret agent mindset too I wasn't doing anything for queen and country it was for my whole family I was 'working'. However, unlike the character James Bond who is never surprised by anything I would react to things rather than anticipate them. Just like the Bond character though at times there would be a certain amount of bravado and even recklessness in the way I interacted with some people. Then there were some days I felt like the world's biggest loser and I was never going to get to the bottom of it all. Throw-away-remarks were very troublesome too but of course to me it was just another comment to take on board. I was like a sponge soaking up every drop of information whether it was visual or overheard. I examined everything, everything that is except why I was thinking the way I was. Of course this is all written with the benefit of hindsight and there can now be the examination or explanation. At the time though I didn't feel disabled or ill, I was not at a disadvantage quite the opposite I had awareness I noticed what others didn't a definite advantage. I no longer felt comfortable at work I was often paranoid whether it was on the phone to customers or face to face with my co-workers.

It isn't of any importance to you what I was 'led' to believe or the conclusions that I drew, that is all personal to me. At the time of me writing this book it will come as no surprise to you that I am what is known as being in remission. Experience has taught me though with each relapse that I revisit my ideas and beliefs so to let you 'in on it' now would put me at risk. Besides this book is in no way meant to plant ideas, be a symbol or signify anything other than my experience of schizophrenia. I have mentioned some things people and events and will mention others but what I believed and believe has to remain a bit vague.

My 25th Birthday was a quiet one which is the way I liked them. Carmen bought me a wristwatch which was very nice it was gold plated the bracelet type with a black face. I got cards and presents from family members too. I still visited Vera and Lorna every so often but with the feelings of being followed it was much less now. I didn't want anybody harming them and certainly not because they are associated to me. My brother Pete had finished with Beth and met and moved in with a new girlfriend named Patsy and as far as I knew she didn't bite. Pete was driving a small van and was self-employed and would do all sorts of jobs. He installed alarms and fitted carpets mainly but light removals and handyman type jobs if he could get them.

It was mid November when Carmen accepted the three bedroom house not far from Vera's and it made perfect sense that I would move in with her and the kids. We wanted to be together and make a go of it and I was head over heels in love with her, in my eyes she was like a supermodel. She had already filed for divorce and had good grounds according to her solicitor. Between us we had managed to get the house semi-furnished and I decorated the lounge and the one bedroom that required it. I remember seeing the double bed in the biggest bedroom for the first time and thinking wow that is for us now. We decided not to inform the social security as it would mean less money at a time when we needed every penny. Apart from getting a new home together Christmas was approaching fast. We found places for the kids in a nearby school and I didn't have any trouble getting to and from work (no physical trouble that is). John Major had replaced Thatcher who had resigned, he was known as the 'grey man of politics'. I began to think maybe things will get better and of course if you add white to black you get grey.

Carmen met me at lunchtime once because we had arranged to have lunch at an Italian restaurant. It was local to work and Liz from the office had spotted us going in. It was not long before we were the talk of the office and then the entire warehouse. Dave asked me to step into his office not too many days later. "So are you two an item then?" he asked. At the time I thought it was none of his business but I did answer, "She is getting divorced and yes we are". He was sat in a chair opposite me and his desk was between us. I could not help but think of Ronnie Corbett as he said, "Be careful because I think you are playing with fire!" I asked him what he meant by 'careful' but he never answered me. "Aren't you scared?" It was as if there were an invisible ball being passed between the dolphins whilst he spoke. I lied saying "Not really why should I be". He said something about her husband being black. "You think I should be scared of him because he is black!" I said with incredulity. "Carmen is black and I am not scared of her I love her". He started nodding and I had visions of the dolphins falling off his face. "I mean he is a boxer isn't he?" He said in a concerned tone. "An ex boxer I think, but for all you or I know he may have a cauliflower arse". I could tell he wanted the conversation to be a sober one but I did make him laugh. It was left with me thanking him for his concern but we were doing okay. "Bloody Crackers!" he chuckled as I left his office and closed the door. I wandered down to the drinks machine telling myself the trophies Brian has could be for coming second couldn't they and then wondered if that was the case for boxers, 'runner up trophies'.

Back in the sales office I asked Liz if she had considered a job with the Manchester Evening News. Nobody spoke to me for the rest of the day in the office it was as if I was being blamed or was responsible for Carmen leaving. The service department was a workspace at the far end of the warehouse below a mezzanine floor that was known as level one. Being sent to Coventry in the office I wandered down there just to see if it was a company wide thing and at first it seemed to be that the three service engineers were blanking me too. Malcolm was repairing a telly, normally the service department repaired electronic typewriters but occasionally they would work on a 'foreigner', fixing something as a favour (and for a price). Account holders were service engineers themselves but very occasionally they would ask the 'Wizard' (Malcolm) to repair what they couldn't. He looked up from the back of the set and said something about a 'black and white' licence. The comment was obviously aimed at me as a titter came from the direction of Albert who said, "Since when do you need a licence to shag". I just said something about jealous workmen blaming their tools and left.

Unlike the office the service department was always deserted during lunch so I made my way down there ten minutes into lunch hour and sure enough they had all gone. Malcolm didn't tend to do much work in the afternoons after having a few pints and would try to get his work out of the way before lunch. I could see he was already behind with his typewriter repairs with three of them still waiting to be repaired. The telly at Malcolm's bench was a colour TV, so then I knew for sure it was a snide comment he had made about the black and white licence. I could see that the 'LOPT' (Line output transformer) had been replaced. There was a small pile of screws and a small glass fuse on the workbench. The only thing I removed was the main 13amp fuse from the plug of the telly. I plugged it back into the PowerPoint which was of course switched to the off position. Then I added another glass fuse, two more small screws, and a small capacitor to the pile. It was sneaky I know but he's a wizard isn't he! I made my way back to the sales office feeling like a very furtive 'Dennis the Menace'.

Carmen and I were getting along great and the kids didn't seem to be too unhappy, we were all looking forward to Christmas. The kids for the obvious reasons but for Carmen and me it was to be our first together. With New Year approaching and a fresh start for us both I knew I could handle anything as long as we were together. The thoughts and feelings were still there but somehow I was not reacting but observing and when I say reacting I mean outwardly, inwardly there was still real fear at times. Not everything I 'discovered' was cause for consternation though because sometimes I would feel that I had a lot on my side, allies, and friends. Even though I hadn't formed friendships it was just a sense of 'we're on your side'. It may have been 'their colours' or things they said not always to me but almost always about me. I would still wear the elastic band on my wrist and would try to stay in the 'Que Sera, Sera' mode of thinking.

I guess anybody who commutes regularly will get to see the same people but for me it was a little disconcerting. Even worse were the new faces of people on the buses or streets. I knew that it wasn't right but especially the black ones and in particularly black youths, but it was definitely not racism thing on my part. I would encounter a lot of dirty looks whilst out with Carmen especially from younger black guys. We both got dirty looks and from all sorts and races of people Carmen seemed oblivious to it though. Even if I wasn't with her at the time it was as if everyone somehow knew we were living together and disapproved. It was starting to feel like the rest of Manchester was holding me responsible for Carmen leaving her husband. I thought we are not just the talk of the company where I work but the whole of the 'Black community' and quite possibly we were the talk of all the communities throughout the country. I was in love with Carmen but I suspected that it was seen as one of my 'moves' or part of my 'strategy' to get involved with her. The truth is I was becoming concerned because she may not be safe her being associated to me. I was wondering whether it was time to confide in Carmen telling her what I suspected was happening. I decided not to though because I didn't want her to be frightened and thought I could protect her from it. Another reason I didn't tell her was that I definitely didn't want to lose her.

My last day of work was on the 21st of December 1990 and I knew I would not be returning in the New Year. I just didn't feel comfortable there anymore and it had all become too stressful. For the past couple of weeks I would only ever answer the telephone if absolutely necessary and I am sure the others in the office had noticed and probably felt they were carrying me. I did however take it upon myself to take on what used to be Carmen's stock enquiry and part identification work. It wasn't like I did nothing but certainly the impetus had changed. When customers asked for me by name there was little I could do but to take their orders. The chitchat and small-talk wasn't the same though I was so very suspicious uneasy and paranoid because after all they were people I had never met face to face. We finished early that day and Dave had provided some cans of lager and other drinks. I hadn't had a drink in a few weeks so it was probably not wise to get stuck in with so much gusto but I did anyway. The firm had the old-fashioned idea of giving each member of staff a turkey to take home. I had drunk several cans of lager by the time Dave handed it to me. "You'll need a big one now you have a family". I thanked him and said something about getting it home on the bus. Apart from the fact that I wasn't that steady on my feet by now frozen turkeys don't come with handles and are not easy to carry. He suggested a taxi but I told him a bin liner would suffice as I didn't particularly want any taxi firms knowing where I lived. I hadn't told anybody I would not be returning after the holidays and didn't plan to do so either. "I'll see you next week then". The dolphins were diving towards the middle of his forehead to indicate it was a question. "All being well" I said. Just as I was about to leave I saw the wizard approaching out of the corner of my eye. "There's a colour TV with all the building rubbish on level one" I said. "It was mine but is beyond economical repair" said Dave. I was slurring my words but said, "It works I fixed it". He looked at me smiling from ear to ear and his dolphins were attempting the vertical trick. "During Lunch yesterday I replaced the 13 amp fuse in the plug". He laughed loudly and said, "You're kidding". I said, "Yes I am", but before the dolphins splashed down I said, "You owe the company 26p for a ceramic capacitor and somebody didn't fit the power supply properly". I didn't know what the hell I was talking about and was hoping the wizard wouldn't ask for details of what exactly I had done to repair the set. I turned and unsteadily made my way towards the half open roller shutter which led to the outside world. I was outside by the time Dave shouted Merry Christmas. "Yes and the same to you too" I shouted over my shoulder. It was the day before during lunch that I went up to level one armed with a screwdriver and a 13 amp fuse. I had heard the wizard tell Dave that it wasn't worth fixing and Dave mentioned getting a skip in the New Year. I unscrewed the plug and sure enough there wasn't a fuse in it. So I put mine in and I just knew the wizard had already fixed it. Not just that but the first thing to check for is the fuse and he must have done so because he had the back off the set when I removed the original. Let's call him Malcolm because a real wizard would have checked again.

The bag containing the turkey was awkward and quite heavy but I managed to get to the main road in one piece. I eventually boarded the bus but on this occasion never ventured upstairs in case I fell down them. I liked Dave and his friendly eyebrows I thought as the bus rattled its way down Oldham Road. The bus was just as cold as the weather outside and I began to wish I had used the toilet before leaving work. It was a ten minute walk from the bus stop to where I lived with Carmen it was dark and getting colder it must have been about half six or seven o'clock. This was a council estate in east Manchester and unlike her last house or my bed-sit most of the houses had gardens. A lot of them also had privet hedges around and separating the gardens. I was dying for a pee and tempted to do one behind one of the trees which were unevenly spaced here and there both sides of the road. It was difficult to ascertain where behind was though as they all seemed exposed on all sides. I decided on this occasion there was no behind to any of the trees and walked a little faster in order to get home quickly. As I passed one garden with the gate wide open an Alsatian darted out and started barking ferociously. I had to turn and walk backwards away from him and it was obvious the fucker would have had me if I took my eye off him for even a second. I was swinging the bin liner from side to side and in front of me as I walked backwards when suddenly the turkey shot out of the bottom of the bag. It landed under the privets of the garden a few doors along from where the dog lived. I was edging my way backwards the dog by now snarling and sniffing at my Christmas dinner. The owner appeared but I never got an apology just, "He won't bite it's alright!" I looked down to where the turkey lay but didn't say a word waiting till he had led the dog away by its collar. I was in desperate need of a toilet and still holding the now empty and damaged bin-bag. I turned and stepped forward but as I bent over to pick the turkey up a pair of pale hands pulled it through from the other side of the bushes. They were high bushes so I couldn't see a thing but I heard a door slam and just as I opened and walked through the gate the light in the front room went out. The bird bandit's house was now in total darkness, I thought about knocking but there was sign on the door - 'Beware of the Dog'. I didn't fancy another near miss experience as I may just have pissed my self. I galloped home like a demented lunatic one hand on my crotch thinking thieves and wild animals were roaming the estate. I reached the house but not the toilet. I had decided to use the grid around the back of the house to save me from kicking doors of their hinges in my haste.

We had a nice Christmas together and I probably over did it with the food shopping out of my last wage but it was worth it. I am like a little kid when it comes to Christmas it still seems a bit magical to me, and people seem to smile more than even on the hottest of sunny days. I like the seaside too which are two of the things that both my Mam and I are exactly likeminded about. It wasn't until after Christmas that I told Carmen I would not be returning to work I had already told her of the snide comments and the tittle-tattle about us. I also told her how they saw me as the cause for her leaving and as if I was somehow a family wrecker. I know most of it was inferred but that was how I saw it at the time. Carmen had just gotten her benefits sorted out and it wouldn't be a good time for me to claim for her and the children. Not just for the financial reasons although we would be worse off but Carmen's divorce hadn't been sorted out yet and it could complicate things.

I decided to go along to the dole and sign on as no fixed abode but they were not exactly helpful. They decided that I had left my previous employment for no apparent reason. I did try to explain that I became homeless and could no longer work as I was living out of a suitcase. I even mentioned the death threats I had received through a relationship and the person knowing where I lived and worked. I know it wasn't all entirely true what I told them but there was some truth in what I said. I say homeless but what I actually told them is that I sleep on different friend's couches and floors and none of them were prepared to let me use their address for fear of jeopardising their own benefits. Like I said not very helpful, I was informed I must sign on every weekday at 10am until such time as I found an address. I was suspended from receiving full benefit for leaving my last job but of course I appealed against their decision.

I soon became aware that Carmen was a telly person she would watch it a lot and not just daytime TV but soaps and quiz shows in the evenings. She would sometimes just settle for whatever was on offer during the day which to me would be like reading one of the shit sheets because it was the only newspaper the shop had. I would try my best to avoid the telly but from time to time I would take on board some of what was being broadcast. I particularly remember a programme she was watching and the presenter saying, 'Just how well do you know your partner the person you live with', 'do you really know them?' I think it was to do with some sort of modern Mr and Mrs Game Show. For me however the questions posed seemed directly aimed at me or I thought maybe they were aimed at Carmen about me. I would notice sometimes that whilst Carmen was on the phone to her mother she would say stuff like, "Yes he is sitting here in the chair". Invariably the conversation would end there and I can only assume that it would be continued whilst I wasn't around. Or she would say to one of her sisters, "I can't talk right now". Apart from my cigarette money I would hand over to Carmen the remainder of the reduced benefit I received each day. I had had to cut down on my smoking for obvious reasons. After about six or seven weeks I was informed one day that my appeal was successful. What I had told them had been confirmed by the company I had worked for and I thought good old Dave. It still meant signing on every day as I had done since the New Year but meant a little bit more money. With part of the back-pay that I received we had a day out in Blackpool. The weather wasn't great but the kids including Lorna got to go on the funfair and it got us all off the reservation for a few hours.

I don't know why perhaps it was the phone conversations (or non-conversations) or sometimes even the programmes that Carmen watched but I began to get suspicious of her too at times. I would wonder just how committed she was to the two of us working as a couple. Our sex life was good and it's nothing I could put my finger on but going back to the questions posed by on the telly. Just how well did I know her, I somehow felt inferior to her or perhaps I thought her family saw me as inferior. Carmen had made friendships with some of the neighbours and their families. I say friendships this wasn't just nodding terms like I had known with any neighbours I had ever had. I would sometimes come back from my daily dole office rigmarole and Deidre her main friend would be sat in the house. I was always polite but felt a little uneasy about her. I found her to be a bit sleazy there was just something about her I did not like. She would make personal comments and sexual innuendos and it was all done in Carmen's presence and more than embarrassing. Carmen had imparted a lot of her personal business to Deidre and her family. For some reason Deidre wanted Carmen not just as her friend but to be their friend too as if Carmen was to be part of their clan. I saw Deidre as riff-raff as for her family and their partners I never knew them but assumed them to be no different.

We were making a nice home together slowly and I had even taken an interest in the garden. I was doing the DIY jobs and not for money I had a sense of purpose and a plan. I was feeling happy and care free some days and suspicious and anxious on others. Sometimes there was that feeling of being invincible and being on top of the world. I was applying for jobs and giving my sister's house as care of address. I wasn't having a lot of luck though some of them didn't even write and let me know one way or the other. I remember some building work close to where we lived gave me access to some free broken paving slabs. I paved the small front garden with them and would buy very small pots of gloss paint that were available as 'testers'. I painted each small slab in all the shades and colours of the rainbow and I suppose this was my very own crazy paving. I would often wonder what the occupants of the police helicopter thought as they passed over our house. I say our house technically it was Carmen's house to the powers that be I was still homeless I had feelings of somehow being caught in limbo.

It was mid April in the evening and just beginning to get dark when Carmen returned home from a hairdresser appointment. She seemed flushed and went immediately to bed and I was left to continue taking care of the children. At one point I went upstairs and she was awake but lying eyes wide open looking decidedly worried. I pulled the blanket back and started kissing her neck working my way down by the time I got to her chest she pushed me away. I know why she pushed me away because just as she did I got the unmistakable smell of sex on her. I didn't tackle her about it but I just knew that Carmen was seeing somebody else sexually and having an affair. She had made such an effort just to go to the hairdressers that morning. She had a bath before leaving and she wore a very smart skirt and blouse suit. The smell I got from her as she left almost nine hours before was the smell of the perfume she had put on. She had been gone the whole day and whilst she was out there was a phone call and when I answered the caller hung up. It was as if whoever it was on the phone was just checking I was at home. Yes it all added up she was two-timing me but who with and why. Then I began to think of the past few months and how long she has been seeing whoever it was. I was out of the house regularly each weekday between 9am and 1pm and sometimes longer if the dole gave me the run-around. I recalled sometimes coming back and the upstairs net curtains were not as they ought to be. They were aside in our bedroom and I made a mental note of it at the time and it was now that I was reading the note. I could only assume that somebody had been stood there watching the entrance to the avenue where we lived. How could she do this to me and so soon, I had made sacrifices, I gave up my home and I had taken her and the children on. I thought about her friendship with the Rutter family (Deidre, her sisters and their partners) I was convinced they were involved in it all somewhere. My mind was racing I was angry and I cannot explain it but sexually aroused too. Just who had she been seeing behind my back and how could she do this to me so soon. I needed some fresh air I felt my face burning up so I left the house telling her to go down stairs with the kids.

Whilst out walking around the estate my thoughts raced I had a million questions but no answers. We were supposed to be in love with each other, I knew I loved her totally. I did feel insecure though because she was so pretty and me so ordinary looking. I thought she was that all time love that everyone seeks but very few find. I passed people in the street and it was as if they knew some seemed to be definitely smirking but how could they know. Maybe I should have seen this coming but instead I am reacting to moves in this game. Yes that's it, it must all be connected she didn't want to do it and they are using her to get to me but who are they though. It still didn't explain how she had met this person though or where. Maybe she had been drugged! I immediately got a mental image of a cartoon like Sweeney Todd character with a hypodermic and a hard-on and so quickly dismissed that notion. No she is lying to me but doesn't realise that whoever it is doesn't want her they just want to get at me through her. She doesn't know about the bigger thing that's going on, Brian must be at the bottom of all this I thought. The traffic seemed louder and faster than normal, I was thinking surely I can work this out then I thought what if it is totally unrelated. I decided I would try not to confuse her cheating on me with the thing I really needed to work out and quickly. I was going to be ultra vigilant regarding her movements and the phone calls from now on though. I would be around a lot more because my sister had recently let me use her address for the DHSS.

She was getting dried after her second bath of the day when I got back in the house. The children were asleep so I shut our bedroom door and I insisted on sex from her. It was as if I needed to re-establish us as a couple but moreover rekindle her love for me if it was ever there in the first place. I somehow thought that I could use my sexual prowess to win her back or keep from losing her if I hadn't already lost her. We had sex four times that night but there was a problem I was ejaculating after just a few minutes on each occasion.

It was the following morning that I was in the bath crying and cracking the backs of the dirty little bastards with my thumbnail. She had given me crabs, how could she and just who was the dirty bastard she had been seeing. I only found four which suggested they were recent, and so did their colour against my red hair, they were brown! The girls were in school and Jerome was at nursery till lunchtime so the rest of that day was to be the start of many heated arguments. She said Brian must have given the crabs to her and I began to think that obviously she had been seeing Brian all along and it was me who was being used. Yes that's it she has been using me to hurt Brian and having no regard for my feelings. Maybe it was some twisted sex game Brian asked her to play and I was the victim. The divorce thing must be a red herring she is using me against him or possibly him using her against me. It all began to actually hurt like having a twisted knot in my stomach. I had to work out if Brian or Carmen were aware of the bigger picture or whether they are part of it. Did they both set me up she would have to be a pretty good actress if she had, in fact she'd get an Oscar. I decided that she didn't know anything and was totally unaware of the bigger thing I was caught up in. Whether Brian was fully aware of the bigger picture I just didn't know. Carmen maintained that she hated Brian and would never have anything to do with him. She assured me she hadn't got back with him. This just led me to believe she hated him because he had given her the crabs and recently. Maybe it was somebody else who she had been seeing but them using Carmen to get to me. Maybe Brian was using that somebody else to use Carmen to get to me. I just could not get the hundreds of notions and possibilities out of my head. In the end Carmen said she had tried a skirt on at Deidre's house and must have gotten them 'innocently'. I didn't believe her and told her so. She tried to say it was me who had given them to her so I told her that apart from her I hadn't been in a relationship in over two years which was true. She had not only been cheating with a promiscuous man but was trying to put it onto my toes. Later that day all the way to the chemists and whilst I was in the shop it was as if everybody was smirking at me.

I handed over the hand written note -

Crab lice, lotion, two people please.

It felt like everybody knew me and Carmen and somehow they knew or expected this to happen. I was never the same after discovering the crabs. There were evenings where neither of us slept because of me insisting that she wasn't being truthful. The arguing went on for days once the kids weren't around we would start again. I am not proud of the way I had dealt with the situation I had destroyed the wristwatch she gave me with a hammer telling her it meant nothing now. I had spat in her face calling her a slut on one occasion and another time I tried to throw the telly through the window breaking a pane of glass and the set. The situation between Carmen and I got worse very quickly it had gotten to the stage where she was saying nothing at all just a blank refusal to discuss things. It looked as though if I didn't accept what she was telling me I would lose her. All along I was still paranoid that the government, MI5 or somebody acting for them was going to do me or my family harm and eventually both things became entwined. I decided that if I worked out the colours, numbers and things said by others in time I would also discover who she had been seeing behind my back. I began to think although she wasn't aware she was to be part of the bigger thing she most definitely was. I even thought that from the day we were both born we had both been steered in a certain direction so that we would meet at that workplace where we did meet. I was thinking that without her on my side I had no chance of getting through this she doesn't love me and I loved her so much. I began to lose interest in everything, food, what I wore, I was going to die soon so what did it matter. I was desperately unhappy I can't do anything right I thought and everything turns to shit where I am concerned. I thought about the last time I saw my Dad alive I was 19 years old and it was two days before he died. I was sat next to his bed in the hospital Pete was on the other side and Vera was there with us. I decided to go outside for a smoke and was trying to get a single match from a full box that he had on his locker. Every match ended up on the floor as I had accidentally pulled the sleeve of the box out too far. He looked at me and the exact words which I cannot forget were - "Can't YOU do anything right, you're fucking useless and you fuck everything up!" I left the ward crying and Vera told me later it was all down to the drugs he was having for the pain. That may well have been entirely true but it's still the last thing my Dad said to me.

Although Karla my sister had let me use her address to receive my fortnightly giro cheque on two occasions it 'hadn't turned up'. Her husband was a big weed smoker and I am convinced he had stolen and cashed my cheques. I am not saying all weed smokers are thieves just that this weed smoker was. It was a bright sunny day the morning I had arrived to collect my giro and it had been three weeks since discovering the crabs. My sister and her kids were out and it was Wayne her husband who answered the door. Amazingly the cheque hadn't arrived! "That's all I bloody need no money again" I said. I thought about knocking him out right there and then and it was only for my sister's sake that I didn't. That day things went from bad to worse I smoked half a joint with him like the stupid idiot I am. Not even ten minutes later I had decided I had had enough and was in his bathroom. It was there that I cut deep across the inside of my right wrist and I immediately felt a tingling and a cold numbness in the fingers of that hand. I managed to hold the razorblade with the injured hand to cut straight across the inside of my other wrist but not as deeply. My hands were over the washbasin the blood dripping rapidly, my life was going down the plughole. My heart was pounding and the tears were welling up because I knew that I really didn't want to die. Not here in a bathroom not anywhere, not yet, why the hell had I done this! The blood was by now a steady flow from my right wrist and dripping steadily from my left. I shouted down to Wayne, "Phone an ambulance I have cut myself". He came up, saw the blood and went to the phone box. I was really panicking by now as the blood was now beginning to spurt and I looked around the bathroom for a towel to stop the blood somehow. It was then that I noticed he used bic disposable razors which were white and the protective cover over the blade was orange. I wondered why he had the old fashioned razor blades on the windowsill and whether they were purposely put there just for me to find and use.

Whilst I was in the ambulance of all people it was Kevin Burnett that I initially thought of. I was in my first ever real relationship with Anne, Lorna's mum. The abuse had stopped and I remember doing some petty very superficial scratches on my wrists after Anne and I broke up. Burnett had spotted them and he said, "Anthony never ever harm yourself over a Woman!" He made me promise that I would never consider it ever again. He was giving me good advice but he was a bad man I didn't understand and it was only now that I really considered it. I thought about Carmen and then Thatcher and I thought about what else he might have said. Once I spent the whole day with him the abuse hadn't stopped yet but on that particular day nothing happened. We were going to the hospital because my Dad had had his second heart attack. Burnett said that there may be wires and tubes and to try not to get upset then he stopped the car. He looked at me and said, "You must find the time to read George Orwell's Animal Farm". I didn't think about it at the time but now I wondered why on earth he had said that and why then. He wanted me to remember it and now I had done. Oddly though whilst reading the book a few years after him saying it I hadn't given it a second thought.

The ambulance had the sirens sounding for part of the short journey so we soon arrived at North Manchester General Hospital. The temporary dressings from the ambulance were being replaced with better temporary dressings in the busy casualty department. It was an effeminate male nurse who gently removed the elastic band from my left wrist. "This one isn't too bad at all but that will not help matters" he said as he removed the elastic band. He did however offer me the band back but I shook my head. I thought by him telling me it would not help matters he must be an ally and have some awareness of what's happening. My mind was still racing as I suddenly became aware of the cameras in the area where I was sitting. I thought about Orwell's 1984 briefly then I thought about my Dad and was he trying to teach me that I ought to treat women the way he had done. I decided that Burnett was there to teach me Chess in order that now I can get through this in one piece but why did he abuse me. By 'this' I mean in order to survive and not die at an early age because by now I was convinced my life was in danger. Was Burnett trying to teach me something else, perhaps I need to be homophobic. I thought poor Carmen doesn't realise she is being used to get at me.

I was transferred by ambulance to Withington hospital where I needed an operation on my right wrist as I had cut through tendons. The sister on the ward was very kind telling me that she and the other nurses were non-judgmental and she put me in a side room on the ward. The wound on my left wrist had been cleaned and stitched and I was waiting for the surgeon who wanted to talk me through the procedure on my other wrist. I was on the bed in the side room hooked up to a bag of blood and my arse was feeling sore from a tetanus jab I had to have. The man who came to see me asked a lot of questions and I assumed he was the surgeon. He asked when I had last eaten, how my sleeping was and did I know the date and who the prime minister was. He asked why I had done it and did I feel that somebody had made me do it. I started to think that he too was clued up or aware of what I was caught up in so was as guarded as I could be with my answers. It was only as he was leaving the room that he told me he was the duty psychiatrist and that he was going to make me an emergency outpatient's appointment. He said, "It's important that you keep the appointment I think you may become very ill!"

When I woke the next morning the ward sister told me that the operation went according to plan and all being well I would be discharged in two days or so. The blood bag had been replaced with a saline drip. She told me my girlfriend would be visiting sometime after 11am Carmen did come to see me and she brought fruit, cards, tuna sandwiches and a portable telly. She set the telly up in the corner of the room and I remember saying that I wouldn't watch it and would have preferred a radio. I was suspicious of what else the sandwiches may contain other than tuna so never ate them. The cards were from various members of Carmen's family but for some reason I saw them as morbid. They were mainly floral and I thought immediately of cemeteries and funerals. Carmen gave me a box of 'Black Magic' chocolates. I had thoughts of her family somehow knowing I was going to do what I had done. It wasn't something I had done myself but something that they expected me to do. I was aware that Vera didn't know anything of what had happened or where I was. Over the past few weeks I had not kept in touch as I felt that she and Lorna would be safer that way. I didn't want her upset and tried to shield her from what I was beginning feel was a huge conspiracy. Carmen suggested that it was now time for me to start using her address and that I should not worry everything will be okay. At the time I believed her, I told her that I loved her and she said that she loved me too. I was discharged the next day with an appointment to have the stitches removed and more appointments would be made to make sure the wrists heal properly.

Carmen had had some kind of falling out with the Rutter family and in particularly Deidre, and I for one was glad they were no longer friends. For the next few days Carmen and I were like the 'velcro couple' I went everywhere with her and it appeared to me that she didn't mind this. I was so very insecure I would ask all the time whether I was enough for her. She told me that she wanted us to be together. I was ever so suspicious of everything and everybody. Carmen had contacted the council about moving house because somebody had daubed white paint on the side wall of our house. She told the council we thought it was racially motivated but I thought it more than that. I was paranoid of every phone call or every knock at the door basically I was paranoid full stop. Whilst we were out in the street the cars and colours of the cars were all mentally noted by me. I even became suspicious of the dogs wandering around and in particularly who owned them. The sex we had was intense but still there was the problem of me coming quickly. I was still undecided if she had ended the affair because if she hadn't I believed she was still being used to get at me but that to her it was just another affair. I suspected every man of being the person who Carmen was seeing behind my back. I even wondered whether it may have been one of my brothers and I asked her. Carmen flew off the handle saying it was a sick thing to say and none of my brothers had ever stepped out of line with her and she would tell me if they ever did. She maintained she hadn't been seeing anyone and she said that the smell on her must have been me from the night before and the Crabs from the skirt. Carmen was like me when it came to personal hygiene so I knew then it was blatant lies because she had a bath that morning of the hairdressers. If she would just be open with me we could draw a line under it and move on, unless it was part of the Tory plan and that's why there's no admission. I decided to just let it drop and observe things for a while but that wasn't going to be easy as it seemed to be somehow intertwined with the government conspiring against me. Carmen came with me to all the outpatient appointments and follow-up appointments concerning my right wrist and hand. After six weeks or so apart from the scars across my wrists both my hands were fine.

Radio news had seemed to change it was quite different in that there was a blow by blow account of events as they happened. I would listen for hours on end it was as though the war was somehow false at times. It was like listening to a drama or a studio production it even had its own title 'Desert Storm'. I became fearful not just for myself but for everybody, future generations, our children and their children. Carmen and I had already started to try for a baby and we had even started to talk about names. I wondered whether it was a wise thing to do but at the same time thought a child would bring us closer together. I told Carmen I would marry her in the future if it was what she wanted.

It was around that time that I received a postcard which read - 'Emergency Psychiatric Outpatients Appointment'. The date of the appointment was October the 19th and the psychiatrist I was to see was a Dr. Green. It was a genuine NHS postcard but it really frightened me. I had forgotten about the duty psychiatrist as it was several weeks ago but what concerned me more was the date of the so called 'emergency' appointment. This was a couple of months away but my 26th birthday would be on the 20th of October and of all the doctors I get a colour coded one! I recalled Brian and the threat about not reaching my 26th I also recalled the 'hearse', his brown car. There was no let up in my speed of thinking and linking one thing to another. It may sound odd but at one point I even considered whether Brian was in some way trying to help me with the threat by somehow giving me a clue. I realised that by cutting myself I had made myself known to the psychiatric people and given myself a history of attempting suicide or harming myself. I had thoughts that if I was killed it could be made to look like suicide. I was constipated so I stopped eating again I had ideas of being poisoned and I would only drink cups of tea that I had made myself. Whilst Carmen and the children slept I would listen to the war news all night on the radio and if I did ever sleep it wasn't for long. I would wake with a start at the slightest noise and some nights I would stay awake to protect Carmen and the kids. My senses seemed acute I opened a tin of baked beans thinking it would help with the constipation and they smelled of pilchards, needless to say I never ate them. This led me to believe that Heinz the company was in on it too, as well as Jacobs and lots of others. The sounds coming from the battery operated wall clock would sometimes seem as if it were as large as Big Ben and louder than the sounds coming from the radio. I noticed everything and for me there was no such thing as coincidence I recalled Carmen saying 'everything happened for a reason'. I thought that maybe if Carmen was setting me up she had gotten to know me by now and maybe switched allegiances. I still had feelings of being on my own and isolated though. I knew what was happening, well not what exactly just that I was going to be harmed but who could I tell. What is it about this girl and why don't I just head for the hills. I felt I was putting her and the kids in jeopardy just by living with her. I thought perhaps it was a case of the black community knowing I was a 'marked man' and they thought I was using Carmen as my shield. It wasn't too long after that I decided to confide in Pete.

I went round to Vera's and I ended up frightening and upsetting her but thankfully Lorna was asleep in bed.

My thoughts were all about Brian harming me because I was with Carmen but I also thought Brian himself was being used. He didn't know it but he was doing somebody else's dirty work if only I could educate him somehow. Pete had turned up at some point and I remember we walked around the estate because I was paranoid about people listening in to what I had to tell him. I was walking and talking at 40 miles an hour telling Pete to keep up with me. At one point he looked at me like he was going to cry but he didn't, I told him I was scared shitless. He suggested I stay with him and Patsy for a few nights. Pete convinced me the following evening that he knew a safe place so it was he and Patsy who took me along to the A & E at the Manchester Royal Infirmary. The duty psychiatrist had a conversation with Pete before he spoke to me. I wasn't privy to what was said but soon became aware of a security guard that had turned up as if from nowhere. The psychiatrist told me I was being taken to Springfield Hospital by ambulance where I would be assessed properly. I had heard of Springfield and I immediately thought that it was the perfect cover to kill a person in the loony bin. There was nothing wrong with me I knew what was happening because I could see the bigger picture and I can't go without a fight I told myself. During the whole time I was at the hospital I was taking in everything that was going on around me. Not just taking it in but feeling that it was all connected somehow to my predicament. Hospital telephones ringing out or other patient and nurse conversations, it was all relevant. I decided to make a dash for safety and was off like a whippet along the main corridor which seemed to be as long as the M56. Closely behind me was the security guard it was as if he had been expecting me to run as I didn't get much of a head start at all. I could here his keys jingling from his belt but I didn't dare to look back because it would slow me down. Now I don't know whether this guy was a rugby player but somehow he had managed to bring me down his arms around the bottom of my legs. I was struggling wildly believing I was really fighting for my life. He had managed to pin me down holding both my arms and pressing my face into the linoleum type floor of the corridor. My nose was bleeding and his knee felt as if it was a heavy anvil pressing down between my shoulder blades. It wasn't too long before back-up arrived and I was carried still struggling for dear life. The two of them were carrying me horizontally I was shouting, swearing, crying and bleeding and I just could not get loose. "Slippery fucker this one" I heard one of them say. The other said, "Yeah, just like that carp I landed on Sunday". One of the bastards' rabbit punched me in the back of my neck and the other one (or it could have been the same one) thumped me in my side. Despite the physical abuse I was still very vocal and quite frantic. I thought it was a myth about padded cells still existing but yes I was taken to a rubber room. There waiting for me was the same psychiatrist from the casualty. "Make sure he's secure now" he told the guards as they carried me in. The doctor said very quietly, "Anthony, this will help you and you'll be able to sleep". I shouted, "How much are they paying you to kill me". Then I felt the sharp needle go into my arse and thought well this is it. They are killing me right here in cold blood and they'll probably get away with it too. I was distraught "Tell Lorna I love her". I thought poor Pete, what a dickhead, hope he is going to be alright. I remember crying and thinking 'Jesus, I hope I am with you from now on'. Perhaps it was a silent prayer and not a thought…

Chapter Four: 'My illness'

I recall being awake in the bed and half aware of where I was but I wasn't ready to let those around me know just yet. I say those around me but as I hadn't opened my eyes I was unsure of exactly who it was around me. The loudest in the vicinity was definitely named George. "Mi name's George Reynolds and I don't give a fuck!" he shouted. He was relating as to how he knew that the IRA had a cell operating locally and every so often would shout and swear. Just who he was relating this information to I didn't know. There was a foreign man who I guessed may be Jewish as he seemed to be chanting quietly. There was somebody else relating the details of a theft to yet another person. I was extremely frightened and didn't know what to expect. Thoughts of how I got here swimming around my head were adding to the fear. George shouted, "Dirty bastards" so loudly that he could have woken the dead let alone me. It was then that I opened my eyes and sat up in the bed quickly realising that my left side and both my arms were very sore. George was an older man with no teeth sat on the edge of a bed that had yet to be made. He was wearing pale green pyjama bottoms and a white vest. I felt like shit! I've had hangovers but this felt like the mother of them all and I had the shakes too. I was paying as much attention as I could to every detail as it could all hold clues for me. I was right about the other man who was stood at the window I could see from the skullcap that he was definitely Jewish. He was middle aged and fully dressed and still chanting and although he was stood up he looked to be rocking backwards and forwards. Occasionally he would look down at the open book he was holding in both palms and for the rest of the time he seemed to be looking out of the window. There was no let up in the Hebrew words if they were actually real words or Hebrew for that matter, I can only say it did seem to flow. I guessed it may have been a Saturday but it was just a guess I had no idea of what day of the week it was. George was still talking about bomb plots but to nobody in particular so I assumed he must be telling me. By now I was aware that it was Richard whose radio and toothpaste were missing and that it was a nurse he was telling. I could only see the back of the pony-tailed male nurse who had called him by his first name. Richard looking over the nurse's shoulder said, "Hey mate take my advice you get out of here as soon as you can". George then shouted, "Fuck 'em all". The nurse turned looked right at me and without telling me his name said, "You look scared". I wasn't sure whether it was a question or just an observation but looking for some sort of reassurance groggily asked, "Well do I need to be?" His response was neither reassuring nor an answer he just said, "I would be if I were you". Or was it an answer! I asked the nurse his name and he told me he was Stuart and that the Doctor would be coming to see me in about an hour or so. The Jewish man stopped chanting and immediately left the room. I got up from the bed a little unsteadily and asked about my clothes as I was wearing only boxer shorts. He told me my clothes were in the locker by the bed. My Adidas tracksuit bottoms and my Man City home shirt were both there and caked in my own blood. My trainers were beneath the bed with my socks in them. I was aware that the bed opposite me had a washbasin next to it and a mirror. I managed to cross to the sink without toppling over but it wasn't easy. The empty bed was neatly made but the bedside locker had no outward signs that it actually belonged to anybody. Stood there in my boxers I looked into the mirror which I realised was actually a sheet of shiny metal covered with thick clear Perspex. I could see bruises on the front side of my upper arms and I just knew they were worse around the back. When I saw my hair I thought white guys just do not suit afros even if they were tidy and mine wasn't. I needed a shave and my teeth were yellow from the chain smoking I had done over the past three days. My nose was sore with dry blood in my nostrils I looked like shit and felt worse. I slowly made my way towards the window walking very carefully it was as if I was on ice but wearing clogs. I was pushing my feet along for fear of lifting them in case I lost my balance. From the window I could see the North Manchester General Hospital and I had to screw my eyes up as the daylight seemed brighter than usual. The windows were the old-fashioned sash type but with wooden blocks screwed onto the sides so that they could only be opened about six inches or so at the bottom. I was standing (just about) on ward 20 on the psychiatric side of the hospital (Known as Springfield Hospital). Looking around more carefully I could see that including mine this area housed nine beds. The ceiling was very high and the paint on it was cracked in lots of places. I asked about a toothbrush, razor, shampoo and soap and I was instructed by Stuart to ask at the ward office. I put my trackies on and edged carefully but awkwardly in my bare feet towards where he pointed. There were no doors it was kind of open plan and to get to the office I shuffled through another sleeping area and again it was all male. It had six beds with one that was still occupied by a man with a gaunt looking face. He was awake with headphones plugged into a small transistor radio. On the bedside locker along with his radio were a half bottle of Coke and a school photo of a pretty girl thirteen or fourteen years old. I assumed this to be his granddaughter as he was well into his 60s. As I passed the bed he nodded in an 'alright mate' sort of way but I never made any response in return. I continued through to the next part of the ward which was the lounge area. The radio was on in the corner of the

lounge a midi hi-fi with only one speaker. The lounge
area was a fairly big space and there were quite a few
chairs in an L shape. There were six or seven people two
of them female and all of them sat down. It was a fairly
Smokey atmosphere so I pulled a flattened 10 packet of
Regal from my right pocket and withdrew one of the
three remaining cigarettes. After squeezing it back into a
tubular shape from a flattish one I asked for a light from
a guy about my age who immediately stubbed out his
cigarette. "You'll have to get one off a nurse" he said. A
30ish dark haired Lady sat two spaces from him said,
"Ere yar love". She had a lit cigarette in her outstretched
hand and I lit mine from hers shakily. I was praying that
I didn't knock the lit end off onto the blue carpet tiles
that made up the floor-covering. I wasn't particularly
bothered about the carpet more what she would say if I
had knocked her fag out. I thanked her as I gave it back
and then sat down on a grey chair with unoccupied seats
either side of me. I wasn't wearing my top but it was
very warm as there was only six inches of air getting in
through the windows. "Have you been sectioned?" asked
the one who had given me the light. "Err am not sure" I
replied. "Section 2 or section 3?" she asked. "I don't
really know". Just then the other lady much older started
to laugh but it was more of a cackle than a laugh then
just as suddenly as she started she stopped. I did notice
that she was tapping her foot which seemed more like an
uncontrollable twitch rather than rhythmic. She was
dressed in a nightshirt and definitely had a varicose vein
problem. From where I was sat I could see the ward
entrance and more to the point the exit. I then realised
that my bed could not have been any further away from
those two swing doors. I wanted to run and escape off
the ward right there and then but my knees felt like jelly
and I was only half dressed with no footwear. Besides if
I hadn't sat down when I did I may well have collapsed
in a heap onto the floor. I started to wonder if the

patients, nurses and doctors were all actors and the ward was like a stage or set. This has got to be down to the government I thought I must have really pissed Maggie off with that letter all those years ago. I then recalled the last pirate radio broadcast I did and thought maybe it had been monitored. I thought in particularly about GCHQ (Government Communications Headquarters). I asked one 'patient' if it was her first speaking part and accused her of being bad at it. It was then that the chirpy morning DJ on the commercial radio station said, "This one is especially for you". He probably said more but that was all I caught of it because somebody was shouting back in the sleeping area of the ward. It was Phil Collins singing his song, 'Against All Odds'. I started to think back over the past year or so my hands were shaking as I put the fag to my lips. I suddenly became aware George was stood in front of me and pointing down at me. "You, fucking wanker you're Irish aren't you!" I never saw him approach but here he was standing over me looking extremely menacing. I felt exposed and vulnerable sat there barefooted and half dressed. I thought I can't get into a tussle with an old man even if I were capable. The Varicose vein lady then screamed, "Nurse!" at the top of her voice. I had to do something and quickly! What I decided to do was move the chair back and away and stand up in one swift movement. What actually happened was the chair went onto its back two legs and I went arse over tit with it. I did a back roll and got to my feet as fast as I could which seemed as if it were in slow motion. It wasn't funny at the time but to an onlooker it would have looked bloody hilarious. Nobody laughed though even the lady with varicose veins remained silent. George was led away by Stuart who spoke to him as if he was a naughty little child. "I don't know what's got into you today Georgie boy". A black guy in his 30s who was seated said, "Take a wild guess, he's paranoid". It was as if it was me he was telling as there was no way Stuart would have heard him say it. "It's all gonna kick off big time a real fuckin' war!" He definitely said to me. I never said anything because I didn't know what to say I assumed he was talking about something in the Middle East though. He got up from the chair and kissed his teeth and the sound was not dissimilar to somebody standing on a prawn cracker. I never saw him again after that so I assumed he only had a small part but at least it was a speaking one. I headed towards the ward office and I could not believe what I saw next. A dark haired young man about my age was walking slowly towards me being led by the arm by a different male nurse. He had his dick out! Not the nurse but the 'patient/actor'. If he was mental and this was a real ward I suppose there were rules about nurses putting patient's knobs away. He was dressed in a T shirt and jeans but sure enough his zip was down and Mr. Happy was out for all to see. He didn't look like an out of work porn star and Mr. Happy wasn't at his best, it was all highly embarrassing. This was like being in a bloody nightmare! What are these people trying to tell me and what does it all mean. It's all for my benefit but are they just trying to make me go as mad as they are if they are mad or have they all been 'resting' too long. By the time I saw the doctor that day I still hadn't bathed, shaved or sorted my hair out. I didn't know what date it was or even the day of the week. I had no qualms about telling anyone and everyone that there was a massive plot to kill me but the killers may be working for somebody else. I was scared of my own shadow let alone the others around me but I thought that if I let as many people know about what's happening or going to happen then it may keep me safer. I was thinking perhaps even if they are all acting in years to come they may feel guilty and spill the beans. If they do succeed in killing me they won't get away with it there are too many people involved and one of them would say something. I thought about Pete and how on earth could he be in on it working against me too, why would he want his brother dead. The psychiatrist who initially saw me couldn't have caught me at a worse time so to speak. He was definitely of Middle Eastern origin and I thought about Saddam Hussein and then the Jewish guy who was chanting earlier.

Eventually I was moved to ward 17 the ward beneath 20 it was a secure ward (locked). It was quieter and seemed a much better environment. I still objected to being there though because I did not feel unwell or ill. I had been detained under the mental health act under section 2 which is for period of 28 days for assessment. Vera visited me with my brothers and I decided they were all in the dark even Pete, there was a row and I told them all to leave. Somehow I sensed they did know something though that I didn't and I would plead with Vera to get me out of hospital and off the ward. It was Vera as my next of kin that had agreed to the section I had discovered. The more worrying section is section 3 which can be used at the end of the 28 day period of section 2. Section 3 of the mental health act is for a period of 6 months at a time and is for treatment not assessment. What's worrying is that in theory a person could be detained for up to a year at a time eventually. Carmen would phone the ward each day and we usually had a longish conversation, she would say that she knew I had something to tell her. For the first few calls it was like she was a priest and I was confessing my sins, I told her all of things I had done in my life that I was ashamed of. I felt so beneath her and unworthy, I felt ugly and her so attractive. I thought everybody that looked at her would be blown away by her beauty like I always was. She came to see me again on my third day there and I asked her straight out whether she wanted to be with me or we could end it here. I told her that she was free to walk away now and I would not hold it against her and there would be no hard feelings. I told her I loved her but that she may be safer away from me. It was one of the few occasions in our time together that she told me she loved me and was in love with me. It was just what I needed to hear because I was still so very much in love with her. She had brought me some new pyjamas and I wondered why it was that women buy new pyjamas when somebody is in hospital. "I have perfectly good ones at home" I said. She smiled and told me that they never cost much as she got them from the market. The pyjamas were grey with white lines on them, I thought about John Major and the government again.

I hadn't been to the toilet for almost three weeks and not for the lack of trying. I was refusing to take or be injected with any medication but I remember asking at one point whether there was anything for constipation. "Yes but are you sure you want to take it?" asked the nurse. "Crikey you're right!" I thought she was tipping me off and therefore helping me. Both Vera and Carmen would bring me cigarettes even so though at the rate I was smoking and giving them away I would always run out. As ever I drank copious amounts of tea but I brewed it myself and I still hadn't eaten. I was having blood drawn every other day from my left arm. I didn't realise it then but it was all about drug induced psychosis and them checking for signs of street drug use. I thought initially it was because they needed to check my parentage. Maybe I am related to somebody famous or perhaps they want to use my DNA to set me up! I eventually got fed up of all the needles so told Morticia and her sidekick Igor to fuck off. Still my thoughts were racing and still I was linking seemingly unconnected things that people had said or I would read. It wasn't until I met Jean the ward sister that I was told that I was safe and not to be afraid. I had been there a few weeks by then though.

I would see a young girl coming back from having electric shock treatment (Electro-convulsive Therapy or ECT). She would be just like a zombie! She was a Black girl of about my age and I thought that she may be there representing Carmen. This person was not only unhappy and confused not knowing what was going on to me it was how Carmen may be feeling. When I say representing Carmen I mean in a way of being used as a representation of Carmen for my benefit. I knew nothing about treatments but it was fear of them shocking me that finally made me succumb to taking Largactil orally. Largactil (known these days as chlorpromazine) is an older drug. The nurse or at that time the person I thought was an actor opened the drug trolley. "Look, Anthony why don't you choose you're poison". I shit myself not literally but he couldn't have said anything worse. "Sorry it was a bad turn of phrase" he said. This is a hospital he told me and we want you to get well, and I don't know why but I trusted him. I was fearful and almost crying though swallowing that first dose. I was having it in liquid form as was the exhibitionist guy. He had been moved onto the quieter ward for obvious reasons. However, his liquid was a brown colour mine was bright orange! It was apparently the same drug though and other patients were having it in tablet form. The fact that I was the only person on the orange liquid gave me a sense of security somehow. I decided orange would be my 'safe colour'. I was given larger doses at regular intervals and sleeping in-between. Sometimes I would wake and my arms were stiff and sore and this was a side effect of the drug. At one stage though I thought I was being injected whilst I was asleep or unconscious. Another side effect was photosensitivity not just sunlight but ordinary daylight too. It leads to redness and irritation of the skin and I was told to apply the factor 25 sun-block that they gave me. Vera had persuaded me to become a voluntary patient and the section was dropped, oddly though I was still on a secure ward. It occurred to me that I may have it all wrong I am not going to be killed in hospital this is where they can't get at me thank God for that. The NHS is on my side and they know I am not a nutter but giving me a place of safety but what if they do think I am mad!

Carmen would visit me every other day or so and we were getting along much better now. Psychiatric wards are not the best of places in which to have a row or let off steam believe it or not. I had decided again that I would try to forgive her and try to draw a line under the whole disloyalty thing. I lied that I believed her when she said she had never cheated on me and had gotten the crabs from a skirt. It was obvious to me that I needed to bring it to a close or it would eat me up. If she had been big enough to admit it though and even if she never told me who it was I knew I could truly forgive her.

I never did draw that line under the affair but I did file it in its own box within my head. I decided that if it was in a separate part of my head I could deal with it separately and not confuse her unfaithfulness with anything else. It is what is known as compartmentalising which was something I had read about once. For the sake of this book I will call that box my 'KISAMO box' (Keep it separate and move on). The kisamo box got bigger over the years and the problem was I always delved into it at the wrong time.

Vera and Carmen both seemed to be getting along famously and I can only guess they had chatted and become better acquainted. They never visited me together but each would speak of the other. Carmen once said, "Don't worry you have got me and your mum for support". Vera once mentioned that Carmen was going to stick by me. My daughter Lorna would send me pictures that she had drawn and even these held 'messages' for me. My fears about dying though were gradually subsiding. Whatever this was all about at least nobody had succeeded in breaking apart my relationship with Carmen or my family. I knew I would not feel completely at ease though until after my birthday. Doctor Declan was to be my psychiatrist and even before I ever saw him he had sanctioned that I got time off the ward. I knew exactly what I was going to do with that hour.

"OK Anthony, no going off the hospital grounds" said Jean. "Are you sure you wouldn't like somebody to go with you?" she asked. "No it's alright I'll be fine" I responded. "OK but remember come back if you get frightened". Jean was one of the old school she had probably been nursing most of her adult life and she reminded me of Felicity Kendal. I imagined her to be growing her own vegetables and hosting neighbourhood watch meetings in her spare time. I crossed to the general side of the hospital which was opposite the psychiatric side. You would think such a large hospital would have plenty of public toilets but it must have been half an hour before I found a visitors toilet near to the new x-ray department. The place was ideal though being warm with toilet paper and it had a good lock on the door. I didn't particularly want to die with my pants down and not on the toilet, and whilst sitting there I suddenly thought of Elvis Presley. Without going into detail I can say I emerged from there 40 minutes later and I was almost skipping. It was like the feeling of getting 8 score draws and winning the football pools! After all it had been close on a month by now since I was able to go. My mood was lifting again I remember thinking if I play it cool I can get off the ward and go home, I had feelings that something had been decided and I had been given a reprieve it's all over. Where was home though was it to be with Vera or with Carmen. I still thought though that maybe the person Carmen had been seeing behind my back has had something to do with it all. I really needed to know that it was really over and that we could try and be there for each other. It was imperative that we stick together because if not I was going to have to go it alone. That would be so very hard though my feelings for her were so strong in that I want to grow old with her.

I was late getting back to the ward and I remember asking Jean whether she thought it was 'a good life'. She said, "Well it can be if you want it to be". Then she said, "How are your thoughts and how do you feel?" I said, "Actually I have just got a load of my mind". She looked at me in a grandmotherly concerned sort of way. "You haven't done anything silly have you?" I had no idea what she could be referring to or mean by silly I just said, "Nope". I told her I was ready to start eating again if there was any orange food. "What do you mean orange food?" She asked. "You know like cornflakes, baked beans or tomato soup but not Heinz". She told me it didn't work like that and that the food is prepared elsewhere. She said she had no way of knowing what would be delivered to the ward. That dinnertime there was no orange food but I did eat though. I opted to eat the food from the foil trays which were sealed. I was told that it was meant for Jewish Patients and as there were none on the ward it was alright for me to have it. I still felt hungry afterwards and recall thinking Jewish food must be like Chinese food in that respect because I had three trays in all. Despite the size of the portions having eaten I felt happier, I had a beautiful girlfriend and life can only get better. I was feeling much better in myself but the suspicious thoughts hadn't vanished completely I still needed to sort things out in my head. I was thinking about all the stupid things I had done in my life thinking back to what Jean had said earlier. I had thoughts of being punished now for something I have done previously and more thoughts of my life and events in it.

It was the following that day that Carmen came to visit me again and it was the first time she had come with the three children. It was the school holidays Chloe, Amanda and Jerome were given drawing paper and crayons. I told Carmen that I didn't want the kids to come to the hospital or see me in here. The exhibitionist guy was in a side room but he was I supposed free to come out of it anytime he wanted. I am referring to him as the exhibitionist guy but with hindsight I now know he was unwell. I told Carmen that if it meant she could not visit then so be it and I said I would write to her and she could do the same. I also told her I didn't anticipate being here much longer anyway. Over the next few days I did write to her and regularly they were love letters assuring her that I was in for the long haul. I would look after her and the kids and I would find work once I was discharged and we had moved to a new area. I must have posted at least ten letters in the first week so obviously sometimes I wrote and posted two the same day. Carmen never wrote back to me but did however telephone directly to the ward each day. As well as my thoughts on the government, MI5, the adverts and signs there were always constant thoughts of Carmen I was so deeply in love with her.

Vera and Lorna and I all ate the cake that Vera had brought to the ward where I spent my 26th Birthday. A psychiatric ward is not a great place to spend your birthday but I felt that there were so many people on my side and looking out for me. I was a voluntary patient on a locked ward and the NHS was helping me. They knew I wasn't Mad and they knew what the Tories and their cronies were up to I just wished that they would tell me though! The nurses let us use a side room which was furnished like any ordinary lounge of any semi-detached. Pete had sent me in some presents, a new Man City top, a radio and some cigarettes. Carmen's Mother Elaine had sent me in some aftershave in a black box with the word 'BOSS' on the box. I liked Elaine although her Jamaican accent was sometimes difficult for me to understand. When I saw the aftershave and the writing upon it, it had me back into the kisamo box and me wondering whether it is all actually connected. I thought about 'dolphin Dave' he was my 'boss' and Carmen's. I thought in particularly about the conversation in the office after Carmen had left and wondered if he was trying to warn me off Carmen. Most importantly I thought Elaine was giving me the answer, it was Dave she'd been seeing and he had given her then me the Crabs. He wasn't concerned for my safety at all he was seeing her himself but was I really that bad at judging character. I decided that if I was then both Carmen and Dave had reeled me in hook line and sinker. I just couldn't get a clearer idea though of where it all fitted in with what by now was a huge plot. I saw Carmen later that day and she looked as gorgeous as ever, we talked a little about getting married again. I thought I would definitely (again) draw a line under the whole infidelity thing in my own head but that wasn't going to be easy even as I thought about it I was considering whether the person she had seen was named 'Bruce'. Then from Springstein (the Boss) it went to Bruce Lee perhaps the guy she had been seeing or still seeing is called Lee. Perhaps Elaine Carmen's mum was saying that it was she Elaine who was the 'Boss' and that she holds all the cards, or maybe it stood for something. 'Back Off She's Sorry' or 'Brain Operation Soon Scally'. I had no control of my thoughts and I couldn't help the way they leaped around and linked things it was as though I was trapped in a puzzle. If I could just find out who it had been using Carmen to get to me I could possibly work out who it was holding all the cards.

I cannot possibly relate everything I felt or thought from moment to moment or even day to day. Not only will it read like you've been slapped around the head yourself but it would run into thousands of pages.

Vera had met the psychiatrist before I ever did. "You've been kicked in the teeth by women and your Dad dying is all part of it" she said. "He also said that you will never be the same again". Pete was with her when she was telling me. "It's Schizophrenia Son". I was stunned absolutely dumbfounded. "It's Bollocks!" I remember saying. I also remember thinking bloody hell so that's what they are up to is it, categorising me as being mentally ill, now I have no credibility. Not just mentally ill but a schizophrenic it couldn't get any worse than that. "You both know it is nonsense don't you?" I asked. Pete said, "Face it our kid you're a schizo". I looked at him called him a cheeky bastard and we both laughed. It may sound odd but if you knew our humour you'd know it wasn't odd for us to find that amusing.

Lying on my bed a bit later on I thought about the whole thing more seriously and ironically being told I was mentally ill just added to my paranoid way of thinking. I can't be mad and not schizophrenia, because I don't hear voices or do bad things and I don't see things that are not really there. I am not scruffy I usually take pride in my appearance right down to my toenails. I am not violent although I can handle myself if I have to which I feel is entirely different. My nature is one of telling jokes and I am a caring person I worry about people, some of whom I have never met. Nope the Bastards used her to get me to where I am now. Who are they though and how did they know she was the chink in my armour so to speak. Perhaps it was all predetermined and I have been set up all along from the day I was born. Then I thought well that's a lot of people in lots of places so I must be pretty important! Then I thought no not important but I have an inheritance perhaps that I know nothing about and somebody doesn't want me to find out. My arse was still sore from my pools win and on and off I had been thinking of Burnett and those first few times. I wondered if he had maybe died and tried to atone for what he had done by leaving me some money or property. If he had I would give it to charity anyway so why go to all this trouble to get me categorised as mentally ill.

Dr. Declan was in his mid 50s and specialised in psychiatry for the elderly so I was one of his youngest patients. From the way he talked I could see he was at home with his older patients. He was a quirky sort of chap as if somehow he'd be reminiscing whilst he spoke. To look at he was a cross between Dickens' Mr. Pickwick and Hollywood's Danny Devito. I entered the room for that initial meeting thinking I would tell him less than was necessary as I didn't want to ratify the diagnosis. "Ah you're a red head, my grandmother had red hair" he said. He motioned for me to take the seat to the side of the desk where he was sat. Before even sitting down I told him I did not hear voices and am not a schizophrenic. "Schizophrenia is an 'umbrella term' you don't need to worry too much about that" He went on to explain that Dopamine in the brain is one of the chemicals responsible for our thoughts. There were other chemicals too they were all known as neurotransmitters.

He said too much dopamine was being produced in my case. "Think of your thoughts as carriages on a steady moving train" he said. "Then it gets faster and faster eventually your thoughts begin to crash into one another". He told me the chlorpromazine (largactil) was slowing my thoughts down and helping me become less agitated. I was warming to him as I knew that since taking the orange liquid I was less anxious of what was going on around me, but it hadn't gone completely. Of course I later discovered that this was just one theory (the dopamine hypothesis) and a simplistic one, I liked the 'train' analogy though. "Okay so that's a symptom of schizophrenia but what is the cause?" I asked. He smiled and said that most patients would say that, that was the cause. "It has never been agreed upon there is an ongoing debate" he said. Then he told me that some think its environmental others genetic and he said the gene or genes hadn't been identified yet though. He mentioned using street drugs can trigger off the underlying illness. "I personally think it can be a combination of two or all of those things". I thought about what he had said and applied it to myself and I began telling him about the cars and their colours when he interrupted, "Well you know at one time all cars were black". I asked about the violent aspect to schizophrenia and some of the other things I had heard. He said if you think about the 'train of thought' again and it derailing. Paranoid thoughts, guilty thoughts, thoughts of persecution etc. all crashing into and on top of each other and yet each new thought along the track still coming. Whatever you see or hear being the basis of that thought but it having a paranoid slant. "Well then you enter psychosis and when people are psychotic and afraid they can act or react violently" he said. "You were psychotic when your brother brought you to hospital". He then told me about 'depot injections' and explained it would keep me well. "A depot injection is an oil based drug that is gradually released meaning fewer injections". He explained that it was better than being on an oral medication because patients can become unwell very quickly. "The drug I have in mind for you is called Depixol". He said it was an intramuscular drug injected into the buttock. "You'd have it once a week to start with then fortnightly and eventually monthly". He told me that we would find the 'maintenance dose' and told me weight gain, lethargy and Parkinsonism can all be side effects. He said there were other drugs for those side effects and I asked whether they had side effects of their own too. He smiled, "Some do yes". He went on to tell me I could remain well saying none of us have stress free lives but stress can retrigger your illness. I thought so now it's 'my illness' that's it then I have been diagnosed now I have Schizophrenia! I told him Carmen and I were thinking of having a child and he told me there may be a 13 percent chance of Schizophrenia being passed on. "Don't be perturbed though having children is everybody's right and 87 percent that your child will be fine isn't anything to worry much about". I asked him whether the medication would complicate things. "Black women generally are quite fertile" he said. Vera had obviously spoken at length to him as he had never met Carmen and I didn't say she was black. He told me to read about Schizophrenia and mentioned the BNF (British National Formulary) this was the book containing information on all the drugs available in the U.K. I had seen 'BNF' spray painted on the wall of the stairs between Ward 17 and ward 20. I thought it was an instruction for me to 'Be NF (National Front)' it caused me a lot of anxiety. I abhor inequality and racism of any kind so imagine being 'told' to change your views in order to stay alive. I told Dr. Declan about the difficulty I had concentrating whilst reading and he said that the Depixol once the level was right would change that. He said that once I had had the first injection the Largactil will be stopped and the time off the ward would be increased. Then I would be discharged as an outpatient to his clinic. It was the longest consultation I have ever had with any psychiatrist or for that matter any doctor. I conceded to my self in my own mental brain that this was a hospital and something wasn't quite right with me. At the same time though I knew there were actual things that had happened running alongside all of that. I did agree to go onto the depot injections and had my first that afternoon all those years ago. I forget the exact dose but it was around 40 or 50 milligrams a week. I spent a lot of the time sleeping and whilst awake was shaking like a leaf which I think was down to stopping the largactil. However, I continued to eat the Jewish food and I had thoughts that the drugs would somehow make me forget everything that had happened. I didn't want to forget though and thankfully I never have. If I wasn't on a list before I certainly was now if not as a radical or subversive definitely a schizophrenic.

Carmen and I started getting a taxi home during my two hours off the ward and as the children were at school quite often we would go to bed. My sexual appetite knew no bounds I was like a dog with two dicks I just could not get enough of her. My sexual stamina was getting a bit better too I was lasting a little longer she may even have had time to boil an egg. Throughout the actual lovemaking I sometimes felt I was still competing with somebody else. I was so jealous of whoever she had seen behind my back it was sexual jealousy as well as plain old feelings of betrayal and hurt.

I remember Pete visited me on the ward on one occasion and I asked him if the chewing gum he was offering me was kosher. He said, "Better than that it's Wrigleys, just chew it Hymie bloody Cohen!" Eventually I did start eating regular food and my appetite was as healthy as it ever was. I didn't interact with the other patients on the ward if I could help it. There was one mixed race guy called Trevor who insisted on being called Moses, oddly he ate the regular food but he truly believed he was Moses. Another odd thing is that occasionally some of the nursing staff would address him as Moses too. To be fair to them this was because he believed anyone who knew or referred to him by the name Trevor was against him. As I discovered when another patient said, "You are not Moses you are Trevor". It was a lot of shouting and swearing mixed in with Biblical quotes and some of his 'own commandments'. He would direct all his anger at anyone who questioned his identity. It was all verbal and although I did not know him I never perceived him as being a violent person just very loud. He spent hours reading his Old Testament and it appeared as if some of the staff had known him a long time. The lovely Jean (shrewdly and yet absurdly) would always address him as petal or flower. I heard her ask a nurse whether any of her patients needed to shower which meant 'Moses' stinks see what you can do please. I could not help myself from laughing sometimes despite the smell which sometimes seemed ward-wide. "Thou Shalt not shower today but have a bath tomorra" he once boomed out to a nurse as if he were atop Mount Sinai. "A fuckin' told ya its written!" They had been trying to get him to shower since he was admitted the previous week. Then there was Martin the older gaunt faced man from Ward 20. The photograph of the teenager went everywhere with him. I discovered it was his granddaughter and she had been killed in a hit and run incident. I once heard him say, "There isn't a tablet that you can give me to make me want to stay alive". On another occasion he shouted, "Does psychiatry have a 'painless death pill' now that would be useful". Martin was on 'one in tens' observations meaning a nurse would check to see he was okay at ten minute intervals. His wife and daughter would visit him every day. They looked totally shell-shocked which is understandable, they had had a lot to deal with. There were other patients and again I decided not to 'get involved' in what was going on for them. I was in my own bubble and they were in theirs and the problems start when these bubbles are burst by either of us. As far as I could tell of all the patients on wards 20 and 17 and there were quite a few it was only Martin and I that had 'get well soon' cards.

Once I was discharged and back home things seemed to get a lot better regarding my thoughts. I was having regular injections so would often be weary or indolent. It sounds like a contradiction but it wasn't always easy for me to relax despite the sedative effect of the drugs. When I wasn't asleep I was often restless and sometimes would pace around not being able to sit down and settle, more in a fearful fretting way rather than an energetic one. I would often go up to bed in the early afternoons because lying horizontally it wasn't as bad and I would soon drop off to sleep. Carmen and I got engaged once her divorce had come through and both of our families attended the party which all went well. I remember it was kind of a dual party because it was Christmas time so our lounge was decked out with the tree and decorations. Carmen told me afterwards that she was three months pregnant and I was delighted.

I saw Dr. Declan regularly and on one visit asked him about me seeking some part time work. He told me not to think about that for now and gave me a sick note. He had written 'nervous disposition' as the reason I could not work (I assumed this to be a kindness). He told me I may well be on medication of some sort for the rest of my life and it definitely wasn't the prognosis I had hoped for. I was having the same dose injections but now fortnightly and he had prescribed antidepressants which also had a sedative effect. I remained well and coped with the effects of the drugs although I was now gaining weight. I still avoided TV and newspapers and still noted the colours (of all things) and car registration plates, adverts and signs. It was simply noting them though and not drawing any sort of conclusions or assumptions. I stopped being too particular of what I was wearing colour-wise.

One night in bed I tried to discuss with Carmen about Brian seeing the kids but it was a very touchy subject. "Do you know where he is because I don't, anyway they don't even want to see him". I thought I will try again at a later date but it wasn't just Brian I was thinking of he must have a mother and other family members.

Carmen the kids and I all went to Pete and Patsy's wedding and it was good to see everybody enjoying themselves. Carmen was five months pregnant at around that time and I was looking forward to our new addition arriving. The people at the renamed 'Benefits Agency' wrote to me saying I needn't send in sick notes any more. This was probably because the last one I sent in given to me by the GP had the illness as 'Paranoid Schizophrenia'. Although the injections were now every two weeks the siesta thing never changed. The city council was dragging its feet with our re-housing application. The term 'loony left' was being banded about a lot regarding Labour Councils. I was pessimistic for the future not just personally but nationally. If there was a scandal regarding politicians it often came down to money with Labour and sex with the Tories. Kinnock really needed to sort things out and I had little faith that he could do it as the Tories seemed to have the media in their pockets. Sometimes I would be lying awake in bed with thoughts of impending doom. Something terrible was going to happen I didn't know what and I didn't know when or why.

In March of 1992 I decided to go to the local library and try and find all I could on mental illness and in particularly schizophrenia. I read a little bit about the life and work of Jung, Freud and Bleuler in one book. Surprisingly they did have a few books on mental illness but none specifically about schizophrenia. I decided I would start travelling by bus again and my first journey was to St. Peter's Square in Central Manchester. For the entire journey I was still noting number plates, colours of cars, colours of clothing and objects etc. it was something that seemed to be programmed into me now. Whilst travelling through the city looking at the billboard adverts and the people it all felt as though it was new to me. I had feelings that I had been in a vacuum and a lot had gone on whilst I was in hospital.

I went into the Central Reference Library to seek advice on what I should read. "If you were diagnosed with Schizophrenia and you knew very little about it what would you read?" Even though I hadn't said, 'I have schizophrenia' there was a sense of embarrassment and shame as I spoke the words. She looked at me as if I had asked where I could find 'Charlie and the Chocolate Factory'. I knew then that I had asked the right person of the three that were at the desk. "I would start off little by little rather than jump right into it" she said pleasantly. "Go and sit down I will find you something". I was walking away to sit when I turned and said, "Oh, and do you have the BNF?" She smiled widely and it was as if I had said something clever or perhaps I had brightened her day. "Indeed we do, yes indeed and I shall bring that too". Over the next few weeks I read all about schizophrenia from collected essays, theories, magazine articles and journals. I read a little on psychology and bits on psychiatry but still not entire books. Dr. Declan was right my concentration did come back but occasionally I would just check the last end word of each line. Sometimes it depended on what I had read in the main text and sometimes it was just something I did before turning the page.

I read that some psychiatrists can explain to patients about a 'chemical imbalance' in a way that has been encouraged by the pharmaceutical companies. The explanation is based on how the drug works and not what is actually happening to the person. I thought perhaps Dr. Declan may have partially done just that with me but still I could not help liking him. I was beginning to get an overview of how controversial and/or unproven a lot of it all was. I didn't want to be 'anti-psychiatry' it is after all a branch of medicine but I could see how easy it would be for me to think like that. I read about Positive symptoms, negative symptoms, 'hearing voices' and hallucinations there was so much for me to cover. Some patients as well as having delusions of grandeur would believe they had 'magical powers'. I also read about the drugs, Depixol for example was allegedly used in the Soviet Union on their dissidents! Chlorpromazine/Largagtil was initially developed as an anesthetic and it can cure hiccups apparently too. I read about 'care as opposed to control' and 'illness and creativity'. Some writers theorised that some psychiatric drugs 'blocked' the chemicals and they didn't stop them being produced a bit like breaking the legs of the messenger. Then there were the studies involving the 'schizophrenic brains' and the normal brains of people at post-mortem. The studies suggested there are marked differences thus there was biological evidence for schizophrenia. However, all the 'schizophrenic brains' had been on various levels of medication for varying years. I read one paper a few days later that said the brain compensates for the blocked chemicals and this itself alters the chemistry of the brain and even its structure. I don't want to get too technical because I am not a scholar or academic but it was all quite fascinating for me. As well as it all being very interesting not having a job anymore it gave me a short term sense of direction. Irene (the librarian) started to bring in articles or leaflets from various mental health groups or organisations and she was really going out of her way for me. Irene was in her late 50s she was a committed Christian and we became friends. I read all manner of things related to the diagnosis of schizophrenia and it wasn't too long before I was suggesting myself what I wanted to read. I would arrive with my ideas and it would be a case of 'bet you have nothing about that!' It was all competitive but in a very friendly way and I think she looked forward to the challenge. Different groups all had their own take on schizophrenia. Ethnic groups, cultures, sexualities, people with physical disabilities and others who had been diagnosed. I also read the history of Bethlem Royal Hospital (Bedlam) in London the world's oldest psychiatric hospital. I even read about mental illness 'treatment' in the Middle Ages which was torture and/or execution, ducking stools, village idiots in the stocks etc. I read that by enlarge it was the church that decided on how to deal with witches or people who were 'possessed'. I read that things were never better with regard to treatment we had come a long way even since lobotomies or insulin comas were the standard treatment. With research into the condition and treatment an ongoing thing I felt a sense of hope for future generations. If my own children were to be diagnosed when they were older at least they had time on their side. I also wondered that if it were genetic why it had skipped so many generations in my case because I wasn't aware of any relatives who had mental illness. I read all manner of things and bus fare permitting I would try to spend at least a couple of hours twice a week at the library researching. I didn't take notes or anything but because this affected me personally I was digesting it all and sometimes I'd relate it back to Carmen. It was after about six weeks or so Irene told me she was retiring and her last day of work was to be that coming Friday. I had just started to read a bit about synchronicity but I decided that that coming Friday was to be my last visit too. With the research and the sleeping I wasn't spending quality time with Carmen and the children.

It was the morning of Irene's last day at the library and I was standing in County Books wondering just which book you would buy for a librarian. The lady at the till looked to be in her mid 30s she had a fake tan and it must have been at least seven or eight gold chains hanging around her neck. "If you had a Christian friend and you wanted to buy them a book they didn't already have what would you buy?" She looked at me as though I had just asked her a question on quantum physics. "A dunno erm did you say dey ad a Bible?" My budget was limited otherwise I would have gone directly to Waterstones. I was about to leave thinking I will pose the same question in Smiths when I spotted it! Of course why hadn't I thought of that it was only April and that will do nicely. It wasn't busy at all that Friday in the Manchester Arndale Shopping Centre. I was sat down smoking in the seating area wishing I had the energy to walk home then I would be able to buy another pastie. I looked at my purchase 'The Friendship Book 1992 – A thought for each day'. I began thinking back to my time in care at the community home.

During week days we would attend classes and it was determined in my first week that I was to be in the top class. All I had to do was read as many words as I could from a laminated A4 piece of card. Classes went from A to D, class A being the 'best class' and D standing for 'dunces'. "You'll be in my class Anthony" said Mr. Saunders. "You don't look pleased it is the best class to be in you know!" Sarcastically I said, "Great lets crack open the champ agney then". It wasn't Borstal but it may as well have been I was so homesick and resented being there in the first place. There was an assembly each morning and each class teacher on rotation would be responsible for a pupil to read from the friendship book. I was persuaded to do this for our class on one occasion. It was quite a nerve wracking experience in front of the whole school (about 70 boys) but as time went on it got easier. It started to be me that did it more often than my classmates. I became a regular reader over the next 10 months or so. Apart from some of the readings the assemblies weren't particularly religious there were no prayers or visiting preachers. Without exception the readings were from the Friendship Book and always started with 'this morning the reading is taken from the friendship book'. I would see the other kids mouthing it as I read and at other times some had started to mockingly say it to me during the day. Occasionally B and C teachers would ask me to do their readings and almost always the D class Teacher would ask me to do his class's reading. The whole idea of the class teachers having a rota was to get their pupils involved. The problem was most of the boys just would not have anything to do with it although there were one or two 'smokers' who read occasionally. I would always do the reading for D class without having to be bribed as I could understand everyone in that class not wanting to attempt a reading. Piss taking and ridicule happened a lot sometimes it would lead to fights. The C class teacher would pass on two cigarettes for me via Mr. Saunders. Cigarettes, tobacco and related items were contraband as pupils weren't allowed to smoke but it was actually the currency of the place. The class teachers were all very different to the 'house staff' with the exception of the B class teacher who thought he was a warder at Strangeways. Cigarettes were also part of Kevin Burnett's armoury in the run up to the abuse.

I was physically shaking I had butterflies in my stomach it was near Christmas time and I had a lot to lose. I had started to get home leave (one weekend per month) and I enjoyed my 14th Birthday with Vera, Andy and Pete so much. It wasn't just nerves but real fear I was embarking on something I knew would lead to pain. I stood there looking down at the open book on the lectern thinking don't do it this is madness! "This morning…" I coughed and looked down at the book and I started again. "This morning the reading is taken from Razzle … and he took her left nipple in his mouth and sucked hard!" I felt like I was a comic at the Palladium the boys mostly laughed, cheered and clapped except for my friend Jay was now standing with his fingers in his mouth whistling. My knees were like jelly I thought I have really messed up now. Mr. Saunders had his hand over his mouth but his eyes were dancing which told me he wasn't cross that I messed up his reading. "Take him to Admin Mr. Mack and Campbell as well" shouted the Deputy Headmaster Mr. Styles. I was led by the arm from the front by Mr. 'Strangeways' Mack (B class). "Take care of B Class Mr. Saunders please" said Mr. Styles. Jay made his own way to the back of the hall. "Classes now please teachers" Styles shouted. It was probably just one of those silly rumours but we all believed the Deputy Head Mr. Styles once worked at Risley Remand Centre. "Quietly unless there's anyone else for the admin block" he shouted as he followed us through the door of the hall out into the cold winter morning.

It was frosty walking across the tarmac of playground to the admin block. The admin block was a building that was partly built on stilts and partly joined to the top of the games room at the edge of the playground. Why it was called the admin block I wasn't entirely sure because on the top floor it was small flats where some of the live-in staff stayed. The first floor only had one small office for admin the other offices were the Headmasters office and the Deputy Headmaster's office. The block was one of the several separate buildings at the home. The others were the four 'houses', the swimming pool, gym and the hall which had the classrooms above. Another rumour that we all believed was that the community home used to be an approved school and some of the staff still worked there from that time. We believed one of the old approved school teachers was the Headmaster and another was Burnett. I wanted Jay to run and I was trying to telepathically let him know that if he ran then so would I. Jay had 'bunked it' (absconded) a few times before, the rule was three times and you were caned. I had only heard that getting 'the cane' was a bare arse thrashing that you never forgot. If I was frightened before blurting out my own reading it was nothing to the way I felt now. I prayed 'please let it be that being a smartarse TWICE in assembly means the cane'. It was too late to run we were halfway up the stairs. Nobody had spoken except Mr. Mack who said, "I will get back to my class now Mr. Styles". Styles said, "Thank you Mr. Mack". We were told to sit on two plastic chairs that Styles brought out from his office. "Don't speak and DO NOT move!" He went through and closed the door to his office. Almost immediately Jay quietly said, "Mad bastard you are Scally". Even quieter I told him, "Shhhh" putting my finger to my lips. I could not believe he wasn't scared he sounded excited maybe the cane isn't that bad after all. After fifteen minutes of silence I whispered to Jay, "Think we will get the cane?" he said, "You kidding, the way they all reacted it's a knocking bet". I asked him if it was really bad and he said, "Bad enough but have never had it off Styles". The phone rang in Style's office and stopped almost immediately. "Shall we Bunk it now!" I said. Just as I finished speaking the door opened "Right follow me". We walked along the short corridor behind him. He stopped at a door and said, "Stand there". He pointed to the wall of the corridor opposite the door of the Headmaster's office. He knocked and then went straight in closing the door behind him. I hadn't heard anyone say 'come in' so assumed the Headmaster was expecting him. I had never spoken to the Headmaster and had never been on this floor of the building before. I had seen him though and of course he had a reputation of being a right bastard whether it was deserved I would know soon enough. They were talking but it was impossible to hear what was being said. Styles came out of the office leaving the door ajar he looked at me then Jay "In you go Campbell". Jay went straight into the office and closed the door. I was stood there with Styles my knees feeling ever so weak. I was listening intently and after half a minute or so I heard the unmistakable 'woosh' and Jay cry out loudly once. Jay came out two minutes later he didn't look directly at me but I could see his face was the brightest shade of red. Styles put his hand on my shoulder and almost kindly said, "Go on son". I wanted to shout 'you know I am a child and you're sending me to be hit' but I didn't.

It was a long room and I had entered it from the side at one end so had to turn. I couldn't give anymore detail of the room as I could not take my eyes off the cane on the desk he was stood next to. "It's Mr. Burnett…" I mumbled. "SHUT UP! unlike your hoppo you are going to be given two strokes". The tears were dripping off my cheeks but I was silent. "Take both sets of pants down turn and bend over and you do not move" he said quietly. He still hadn't moved from the side of the desk at that end of the room. I did just as I was told my arms were stiff and my fists clenched. "Now put your hands on your knees" he said and again he spoke quietly. I could see my laundry number '31' written in black ink on the white label which was stitched into my trousers. I heard him do a practice swing of the cane and closed my eyes. He ran from where he was standing I didn't hear the woosh but it felt as though somebody had placed red hot copper wire across my arse. I screamed as I hit the deck with my eyes shut tightly I went into the foetal position on my side curling up as small as I could possibly get. I gasped in the air in order to cry out again when I felt the pain across the outside of my right thigh. I thought I was going to black out when he gave me another whack this time catching my right forearm. He said two but gave me three and yes he deserved his reputation for cruelty and more. I was on the floor screaming my heart out with my pants around my ankles. He never spoke but left me to cry and it must have been a good five minutes before I stood. I pulled my underpants up and my trousers I was still sobbing and sniffing. I fastened my pants and turned he was sat behind the desk and still he didn't speak. I wiped my eyes which seemed to be stinging I looked down to that end of the room. His eyes were closed and all I could see were his grey eyebrows and pale eyelids. With his eyes still shut he pointed to the door so I left the room. "You're mate cried too Scally" said Styles as he handed me several tissues. "You're to stay in your room the rest of the day and the housemaster will see you get your meals". This guy knew that this was abuse and it was wrong I could tell from his voice. I blew my nose loudly and I saw him look directly at the now swelling thin red ridge across my forearm. "You can't go home at weekend for three months". I wanted to cry my heart out again and scream the place down, "Bastards" I said croakily. He pretended he hadn't heard and gave me the good advice of not having a bath for a week or so.

My peers saw me in a different light after the 'Razzle' incident, the sexual abuse stopped and I knew I had a true friend in Jay. Corporal punishment was abolished by the time the school became mixed in 1980 and it was at that time I met Anne Lorna's mum..... I looked at my watch and it was almost 1pm I took a biro from my pocket and the Friendship Book from the carrier bag and I inscribed the book.

Chapter Five: Under the umbrella

My son Ashley was born in July 1992 and by the end of that August we had accepted a new four bedroom house. The council house was in South Manchester and right opposite a primary school. Chloe, Amanda and Jerome soon got places and we put Ashley's name down for when he was old enough. I received a letter around that time from Margaret Warburton who was to be my Social Worker. I hadn't had a social worker since my latter days in care and overall my experience of them was good. I could only assume that South Manchester had the resources that North Manchester didn't but was glad Dr. Declan had written to Margaret. I liked Margaret straight away she had empathy and consideration but not pity. She was highly professional yet unassuming and caring she became more like a friend of the family than a social worker.

I decided that the model for our household and raising the children would be like that of the family group home where Pete and I spent some time. This in itself wasn't always going to be easy on a budget made up from state benefits although we were not as badly off as some people. Carmen started to take driving lessons it was £10 per hourly lesson and we could only afford two lessons per month. I had decorated the house a room at time and we were furnishing the rooms, again a bit at a time. Margaret would phone every few weeks and every so often pay us a visit she only worked part time and was looking to retire soon. Margaret was well travelled and had visited lots of places all around the world, each time she came to see us we'd enquire of her next trip.

I would try and make the journey across Manchester to see Vera and Lorna whenever I could. Vera was a bit worried as Anne Lorna's Mum had recently returned to

Manchester from London. Lorna was starting to hint at wanting to live with her Mum once her Mum found somewhere permanent to live. Lorna was about to start high school and by all accounts was doing really well at school. Anne hadn't really learned any parenting skills which was Vera's main worry. My brother Pete and his wife Patsy had managed to acquire the lease of a carpet shop in East Manchester. Pete was enjoying working for himself and the handyman type jobs had become less important to him with carpet fitting work taking priority. Pete and Patsy were looking to start a family but due to medical issues Patsy couldn't conceive naturally, so they were accepted onto the IVF programme at St. Mary's Hospital. I kept in contact with Vera on the telephone most evenings and had a looser contact with Pete.

It was a Dr. Breen who was to be my new psychiatrist and my first impression of him was good too. Dr. Iain Breen was erudite yet with the common touch I felt. He was softly spoken with a slight Scottish lilt in his voice which seemed to convey a kind of equanimity. I decided I was going to get my life moving in the right direction and get the medication down to 'maintenance dose'. Things weren't as bad now though as when I was on the antidepressants (Surmontil) during the previous year. It may sound odd antidepressants and feeling bad but they had sedative properties and I felt like I was sleeping my life away. I often wondered how the unpleasant side effects of the drugs can be good for ones mental health and that is why I needed to get my level just right. It wasn't just the lassitude, Parkinsonism, erectile dysfunction, constant dry mouth or muscle stiffness but the medication somehow also impeded my momentum for life itself. I believed I could get the Depixol down even further after all I could refuse to have any drug at anytime if I wanted to but as bad as it was for me there was no way I wanted to feel as frightened as I had done in 1991. I also wondered whether maintenance dose would be a 'comfortable dose'. I was hoping the 40 milligrams every two weeks wasn't going to be seen as the best dose for me. I wanted to get back into employment in order to provide for Carmen and the children.

I was seeing Dr. Breen regularly and sometimes took part in studies and/or research at his invitation. I would be paid £5 for my time from some fund or other. I was happy to help whether it was for students or other Doctors and it got me a packet of fags. South Manchester University Hospital Trust is a teaching hospital and as the name suggests is linked to the university. The psychiatric wards and psychiatric outpatient clinic were all based at Withington Hospital and there was also a 'Day Hospital' on the same site. I hadn't broached the subject of medication with Dr. Breen yet because he was aware from our consultations and my notes that I was taking Largactil again. I had it in tablet form but only in small (but regular) doses, Dr. Declan had suggested it as a short term measure when I came off the antidepressants. So I thought the first thing I must do is get off the orals before even talking about the depot injection being reduced. I remembered from my research that I had read about some drugs being prescribed 'PRN' (from the Latin 'pro re nata') basically it means 'to be taken if needed'. So I decided I would discuss with Dr. Breen about using the chlorpromazine PRN and see how I got along.

Our first Christmas at the new house was a good one I even managed to sit through a couple of the films shown on telly without becoming overly anxious. Carmen and I were getting into petty arguments over silly things though so in the New Year I mentioned it to Margaret. She suggested perhaps we were together too much of the time and asked if I would like to go to the day hospital from time to time. In the February I discussed it with Dr. Breen on one of our outpatient appointments and he thought it would be a good idea too. To my surprise at the same time I negotiated a reduction in medication quite easily but it wasn't the orals. The frequency of the Depixol would now be every four weeks the dose of 40mg wasn't changed but it was of course a reduction of the amount that would be in my system. I still had to take the chlorpromazine 10mg orally twice a day but I was pleased that I may be able to function better from now on. Things were looking up as Carmen had passed her driving test and we had bought a second hand car. I was so proud of Carmen for passing her driving test on only her second attempt. The car a sky blue Austin Maestro we nicknamed Ethel.

It was early April 1993 I was up and dressed earlier than usual as I was to go to the day hospital for the first time. I received two items and a letter in the mail on the same day. The letter was from Disability Living Allowance I had been awarded the 'middle rate for personal care' it was just over £30 per week and awarded for 'life'. I also received a free bus pass that allowed me free travel on any bus, train or tram within Greater Manchester. The other item was a CD of 'The Three Tenors' a free gift from a music club I had recently joined. I thought about the CD and the 'three tenners' a week I would be getting from DLA and couldn't help but smile. I had Margaret to thank for the pass and the DLA and I did thank her when she picked me up to take me to the day hospital a bit later that day. Margaret only took me that first time after that I would make my own way there on the bus.

I had agreed to go to the day hospital on week days in the hope that it would add structure to my day. Now that it didn't cost me anything if I felt anxious I would get off the buses more often and would wait for the next one. Occasionally Carmen would take me to the day hospital or pick me up from there in Ethel the car. The day hospital was a very good resource for those who needed it but unfortunately I soon began to feel that I could manage without it. Smoking and drinking tea all day is something I could do at home, but to be fair other activities did go on too. I never got involved in the day trips because if travelling by car I would always have to sit next to the driver. The day hospital had the use of a minibus for the day trips and the nursing staff would always sit up front. Each day at various times medication would be given out and some people would actually start to queue up for it early. I was given one of my 10mg chlorpromazine doses this way but I was never known to queue for it. I often felt it was unnecessary as I was perfectly capable of being responsible for my own meds. It was from the same 'meds room' that I would collect my factor 25 sun-block every two weeks. After a few months I realised the day hospital wasn't really my cup of tea I had tried occupational therapy there and one of the art groups but none of it suited me. I know lots of people did enjoy the lessons or OT but to me the pace and atmosphere just seemed like being in primary school or even a nursery at times. There was a certain amount of apathy from the mental health patients at the day hospital perhaps it was partly their illnesses or perhaps their medications. I felt luckier than most that my levels of meds were smaller in comparison but I still wanted it reduced further. There didn't seem to be any debate, topical discussion or laughter even, at least not that I ever noticed. A lot of the 'service users' seemed to have assumed the 'sick role' and saw themselves as victims. Of course they have every right to feel that way if they wanted to it was just that I didn't want to feel like that.

I remember seeing SMUG written on one of the office doors in the corridor at the day hospital and was told it stood for South Manchester Users Group. Apparently I was a 'user' which is short for 'service user' unless I was on a hospital ward then I would be a patient. Initially I thought about the same term 'user' being coined for people who 'used' street drugs. I suppose if people lived in the community then they couldn't be patients so user (or service user) seemed to fit nicely. As for 'smug' I saw that as being a rather unfortunate acronym it couldn't possibly have been intentional.

Sometimes I would smoke, drink tea and play cards in the ATU (Alcohol Treatment Unit) which was a separate unit but on the same site. I got to know some of the service users on the unit and the atmosphere there seemed more friendly and buoyant. They all knew I was from the mental health side of the hospital and it didn't seem to bother them any. One Scottish guy Graham would often shout in a broad Glaswegian accent, "Scarrrlly is it a schizo ye are!" Invariably I would respond with just the one word - "Allegedly!" I would place a regular order for 'duty free' hand rolling tobacco with him which I smoked between packets of regular cigarettes. Now the ATU was just a place to smoke and drink tea for me and I suppose for the ATU service users it was a better option than being in a pub drinking and smoking. They also had groups and sessions relating to alcoholism but of course I didn't participate in those. As the weeks went on I decided I needed something else to structure my days ideally I need a proper job.

I spoke to Margaret about not finding the day hospital worthwhile and she suggested referring me to an organisation called 'Options'. Options were like a job agency with government funding, getting people into (or back into) employment or training. Their service users were people with learning difficulties but they were looking to include people with mental health problems. At my initial interview with options in August 1993 it suddenly dawned on me how difficult it is going to be to get back into 'mainstream' employment.

Parminder was a softly spoken Indian gentleman responsible for assessing potential service users for Options. "Schizophrenia, wow what is that like?" he asked. I thought for a moment and said, "Well how long have you got?" He smiled but said nothing as he was still waiting for me to answer. "I have good days and not so good days" I said. I mentioned the medication, the side effects and some of the actual issues that led to me being diagnosed. "You do realise that if you are placed with an employer or in training we have to disclose your diagnosis" he said. He told me that it was also the case if asked about existing medical conditions on any application form or at any interview. "And if I didn't mention it what then?" I asked. "We have to mention it but if you find employment independently and don't mention it you could be sacked on the spot if they find out". I thought about what he was saying and I told him it was like having a criminal conviction. He nodded and went onto say it was the same with insurance companies if I ever wished to drive. He suggested that I could do three days a week to start with at one of the options offices in East Manchester just until they found me something permanent. I lasted just under two months it was okay at first but in the end I realised it wasn't the stepping stone I had hoped for. It just wasn't worth it for me, not just the stress of travelling across Manchester but once at the offices there was little for me to do. The only plus about it was that whilst in that part of Manchester I would visit Vera and Lorna. There was another service user at the options offices whose name I don't remember she would empty litter baskets from the small staff offices that were behind the reception area. She'd make tea and take orders for sandwiches etc. at lunchtime. I couldn't get involved in any of that otherwise she would have had nothing to do. There was a computer room with printing facilities but on the days I was there it was never used. I asked permission to use a computer for word processing and was told that it would be okay. The only thing I recall writing was -

'Having the diagnosis of schizophrenia is just as traumatic as the illness itself.'

It was to be the start of an essay but I never got beyond the first few lines I would sit for ages just looking at the screen. I spent most of my time just playing card games on the computer. Occasionally I would open programs or applications just to see if I could get the hang of using them.

One morning shortly before I left Options the outside agency worker Linda had called in sick. Linda worked on the reception desk and we got on very well, we would have our fags together outside at various points through the day. I would tell her of Ashley who was now beginning to toddle around and would talk all about Lorna, my step-kids and Carmen. She would relate about her loved ones too particularly her boyfriend Mark. Linda was about 23 and a graduate doing temporary work and she was about to relocate to London with Mark. There was a mix up that morning because the agency that had placed Linda with Options didn't have anyone to cover for her. I offered to cover for Linda telling the members of the options staff that I could probably take calls and messages if somebody showed me how the phones worked. By about 10am I had sussed it out completely there was nothing stressful about it and I was entirely confident. I was putting people through if the staff wanted to take the call and taking messages if they didn't or were not at their desks. I was letting staff know when people presented themselves to reception and offering/making drinks whilst they waited. It was the best day I had had at options in the seven weeks I had been there. At one point I handed a message slip to one of the members of staff and she commented on how I was doing a terrific job. As she took the message slip from me I noticed her eyes as she saw my tattoos. "I am not sure if you could work on reception permanently though, dealing with the public face to face". I just said, "Oh alright". In all the weeks I was there Parminder had still not managed to persuade even one potential employer to give me a chance.

It was a conversation with Linda that brought home to me what the average person thinks of 'people like me'. I had only ever mentioned 'mental health problems' to Linda and she had never directly asked for more information. She must have assumed that I had some form of depressive illness as my outlook at times was very pessimistic in particularly with regard to getting work. I was having a smoke outside with Linda and we got onto to the subject of mental health and employment again. "They'll find a placement for you soon don't worry it's not like you're a schizo or anything". I didn't enlighten her but discovered that she held some firm beliefs about people diagnosed with schizophrenia that were totally wrong. I couldn't blame Linda as I had assumed all of those things myself but that was before I was diagnosed. I felt slightly pathetic not challenging what she said or even admitting that I was actually one of those people she was talking about.

I was one of that group of people at least, but surely every person is unique it's not like we have all been cloned or had become doppelgangers.

I thought back to when Dr. Declan said that schizophrenia is like an 'umbrella term' and I needn't worry about it. I was worrying though because I didn't want to be a 'schizophrenic' and I didn't want to feel ashamed if the diagnosis was right. I felt that the whole problem with the 'umbrella term' was about some of the others that were under the umbrella with me. I never went back to options after that and I became despondent, my life, my situation and my future all seemed so hopeless.

I agreed to go back to the day hospital but it was when I felt like going rather than regularly or routinely. One of the quietest spaces at the day hospital was the non smoking area facing the nursing office. The chairs were comfortable and there was a certain amount of privacy. The area had several screens or room dividers something like the Japanese have in their rooms. The screens were painted to look like orange trees and you could almost imagine being in an orange grove at times. I was sat there contemplating on where I could go for the day because as I had free travel I thought I may as well make use of it. "I'm a schizophrenic are you?" I looked up and it was one of the service users I had seen around the hospital. He sat down on the chair opposite me and there was a small low table between us. "Well are you?" I thought about using my standard reply of 'allegedly' but then felt I needed to educate him. Educate not in a condescending way but I didn't really want him to refer to himself as a 'schizophrenic' and certainly not introduce himself as one. "The doctors say I have schizophrenia but schizophrenic is not something I would call myself". He asked me whether I believed in God and whether my voices were God and God's son Jesus. I told him I didn't hear voices and I was undecided on the whole religious thing. "Do you know Dave Woodley?" he asked. "Who does he play for?" It irritates me when conversations are all about whom we know and how we know them. It's like the person mentioned has somehow managed to invade, monopolise and impose themselves into the conversation without even being there. "He doesn't play football he's a hard twat, you must know him, I do we're good mates". I told him I had never heard of him but that it wasn't surprising as I keep very much to myself. My thoughts of educating this guy changed to thoughts of wanting him to go back into the main smoking area. "Ever fucked a thirteen year old virgin?" I wanted to say that thanks to people like him people like me had to endure a sense of disgrace but I never. "Was it God or Jesus that just heard you say that?" He didn't answer. "If you don't hear voices then you are not really a schizophrenic" he said. I asked him whether that was his professional opinion or something his own voices told him to say to me and I reminded him I wasn't a 'schizophrenic'. "Where do you live?" I was in no mood to continue talking to him he had come along and upset my flow whilst I was minding my own business. "Not far, listen you're annoying me can you go away please". He clenched his right fist and wrapped his left hand around it. "Do you want to know where I live?" I told him that I didn't particularly want to know and that I already had an idea of where he lived. "You're not even a patient you're staff pretending to be a patient". I told him I was a service user just like him and all I wanted was to be left alone. "Okay just tell me one thing and I'll go, where do I live?" I looked at him and said, "Doppelville!" He smiled showing his crooked yellow teeth and told me I was wrong then he stood and purposely kicked the table that was in front of me. Obnoxious bastard I said to myself as I watched him disappear onto the corridor which led to the other lounge.

Now I know that this guy had been diagnosed with schizophrenia but I felt I couldn't make allowances because of it. To me it would be like all white people saying racism was okay against black people because the racist was white or vica-versa. Or if the guy was a racist (and it would not surprise me) it would be like saying it was excusable because he has schizophrenia. Now there are plenty of racists and people we may find obnoxious walking around but this man to me was using his illness to frighten people. I was prepared to put money on the fact that he didn't speak to his psychiatrist the way he had just spoken to me. However, the phenomena of 'hearing voices' and the fact that he wasn't the brightest button in the box also made me wonder if I was being overly intolerant.

"There but for the grace of God go I". It was Bill Morris one of the nurses. He knew me quite well and we had talked on many subjects including schizophrenia. "We are all chemical factories you know Anthony". Bill had seen the service user kick the table as he left and he reminded me that it was almost time for the user's meds to be given out. "What's being a chemical factory got to do with it?" I asked him. He explained that the brain is so complex in particularly thoughts which can affect our behaviour. "You know adverts with catchy songs?" He looked at me a little bemused. "Well they stay in your head for ages" I said. "Yes" He nodded. "And sometimes when you see the product the song pops up again". He started smiling. "Do you think they are trying to alter our brain chemistry to buy the product or something more sinister?" He laughed then said, "It's all about the product and if they are trying to alter brain chemistry I personally don't think it works like that". So I asked him how he can excuse what he himself had called 'learnt behaviour'. "Now you know very well that I think it's more than just that Michael's mother is mentally ill too". We had never discussed religion but I got the impression Bill may have had a faith and he seemed to be thoroughly wholesome and I liked that about him.

Chapter Six: Freed To Kill

Carmen was driving straight down the middle lane of the motorway we were on our way to North Wales. It was the half term holidays and the Social Services were paying for us all to spend four days at a holiday camp. It was something none of us had experienced before and I had thoughts of it being something like the TV programme Hi-de-hi! I was being hyper critical of Carmen's driving and in particularly her not using the inside lane. "You can't even drive so don't start all that" She told me. I could see the other drivers flashing as they passed us some being forced to undertake and I could see they weren't happy. Not wanting to have an argument and spoil the excitement of the day for the kids I said nothing more. It was a great four days and although the facilities were not exactly five star and it was a budget chalet it was all clean and the people friendly. The kiddie mascot was a crocodile and I forget what camp catch phrase was but it wasn't Hi-de-hi. The weather wasn't that great it being October but there was an indoor swimming pool, a few play areas for the kids, a bar and the main entertainment room. We had a terrific time doing the usual things, we played prize bingo, took part in family quizzes and watched family cabaret. It was during the break in one of the shows that I was propositioned in the Gents toilets! When I got back to the table the kids were playing on video games so I told Carmen and she found it highly amusing. I began to think back to the period before I moved into the bed-sit in the high rise block. I was doing some decorating work for somebody for £30 and met a guy through that person and he gave me more work at his house. To cut to the chase I became involved in a ménage à trois not in the classic sense of living with him and his wife and not the fact that I had any sexual contact with him. He always referred to it though as a ménage à trois but he was actually a watcher. He would 'direct' as if he was Spielberg but it was only for his viewing pleasure and not filmed. There was a lot of role play and he would set the scenario he would give instructions both before and during the sex. I was paid at first but in all honesty once I got over the initial first awkward and amusing couple of times I would have done it for free. Then he told me that he was getting too jealous for it to continue and I thought he meant jealous of me with his wife. He actually meant he was jealous of his wife with me. He propositioned me and for the next few months I was involved in a homosexual relationship with him. It was all surface and it never went beyond mutual masturbation or him watching me, despite his insistence for more than that. There were gifts, love letters, cannabis and days out whilst he was on strike from work. It was all very flattering but I needed to get out of the relationship it wasn't what I wanted and I told him so. He had a wife and a daughter my age and I couldn't buy that best of both worlds crap because that's how people get hurt. Although I never mentioned Burnett he even used the 'don't knock it till you've tried it' bullshit on me. I did get out of the relationship and the last time I saw him was when I got out of his car, but the trouble was it was still moving at the time. It was another of those arguments all about what he wanted and him putting pressure on me to be 'his lad'. "Just fuck off out of my life and leave me alone" I said as I jumped out of the passenger door. He turned the car around and driving slowly alongside of me he continued to harass me pleading for me to get back in. I told him if I ever saw him again I would contact the police and assured him I would speak to his wife and daughter. I probably wouldn't have done because he was basically a nice guy but I never did see him again. I limped home and was off work (YTS) for two weeks with a badly sprained ankle. When we got back from our holiday Carmen and I agreed that we would go on holiday as a family once a year for at least one week.

In November I went to a local church just to see if they had anything organised for bonfire night. It wasn't a catholic church and why I thought any church would celebrate or commemorate the gunpowder plot I don't know. They didn't have anything planned and were in the middle of painting one of the halls of the building, they invited me to grab a roller and get stuck in. I decided not to get involved but found everybody friendly and took them all at face value. The Minister was the Revd. Andy Knight and I had already seen his wife Angela before as she was one of the local lollipop ladies. I was told everybody was welcome at the church whether that was on Sunday's or weekdays. I spoke to Carmen about us going as a family to church and that is what we started to do each Sunday and I began to think that there were some nice people on the reservation after all.

Christmas was quiet and I couldn't have wished for a more wonderful experience I had everything I wanted. A family of my own our house was nice and we had a car but it was much more than just the material things. If only I could get a job then I would be able to answer those questions like 'what do you do?' or 'how come you don't work?' I knew that if there was such a thing as a job that was 'Anthony Scally Flexible' everything would be perfect, a job where I was able to walk out at anytime if there was anxiety or paranoia. Nobody has the perfect job though especially one where you could go for a kip in the middle of the shift. It would have to be a job that didn't involve too much interaction with other people and what if I became ill again. The disability benefit system worked on a Ladder scale of the longer you are in receipt of incapacity benefit the higher rate you eventually got there was of course a ceiling. I didn't send in the sick notes anymore so was classed as disabled and was on the highest rate of benefit. The problem was that if I came off benefits into employment and was then unable to work again due to a relapse I was back on the bottom rung of the ladder. This is why employers asked the questions about pre-existing medical conditions because they didn't want to pay somebody long term sickness pay. Whether it was also partly a case of not wanting somebody diagnosed with schizophrenia working for them is debateable. I began thinking I would look for flexible work and I would not disclose my diagnosis. If I did become ill as far as they were concerned it would be the first time or 'first episode' of illness but that would mean lying. In the end I felt it was all too much of a risk for the family and I thought not only was I caught in the benefit trap I was unemployable. The solution was found when Carmen said that she would go back to work and that I could take care of the kids and our home. I looked into claiming for me and the kids and that is what I did and of course I kept the DLA.

In the New Year of 1994 I became a modern man a 'stay at home father' I was a househusband, or what these days is called a homemaker. I didn't have to assume the sick role and if anybody asked I had something to tell them other than 'I don't work due to disability'. Carmen got secretarial work through various agencies and the work would usually be in the early evenings, during the days she attended college doing computer literacy. Cleaning and cooking etc. was something I had always been involved in at our house so it wasn't anything new. Taking care of the children wasn't new either as I had done that before although now I didn't have Vera to share in the responsibility. Ashley had started part-time in the nursery class at the school just over the road and usually by lunchtime my work was done. Ashley would sleep in the afternoons and so would I and I don't know why but he had a way of waking up that always gladdened my heart. He'd go from a dozy sleepy state to a gradual wide awake bright-eyed 'hey here I am now give me your full attention'. Looking after things domestically wasn't seen by Carmen as solely 'my job' as she did her share when she wasn't at college. There were still thoughts about colours and things seen, heard or overheard but all of that just seemed to be inbuilt it wasn't intense and I never reacted. Margaret would visit now and then and we talked on many subjects she often commented on my great 'insight' into my illness and my personality in that it hadn't become flattened. She commented also about my sense of humour and I said that I wished she had known me before I was on medication. Occasionally she would bring a student or colleague and it felt as if she was showing me off but in a way that she wanted them to see me as an individual. At that time though being unique is one thing but I hadn't met anybody in my situation diagnosed with schizophrenia but feeling that it was undeserved and political or me knowing too much and seeing the bigger picture.

Even as I write I think that may also still be the case so if I am found dead or die an unexpected death perhaps what I have written will make people stop and think. At the moment being harmed doesn't scare me but there are times when it does and there are other times when I think my kids will be harmed. I could write for hours about my thoughts that there are a handful of people that control the world and they are not the 'world leaders' that we all know and have elected. I could write about how advertising isn't as it all seems and consumerism will 'eat itself'. The purpose of this book is to relate the events and my thoughts as they happened and I accept that to the rest of the world my way of thinking means I have mental health issues. I don't want to write a conspiracy theory or other such rant that isn't the purpose of the book. It's banded about a lot but 'just because you're paranoid it doesn't mean they're not out to get you.' I want to help others, help the medicos and I want my children to know how dad came to be diagnosed with schizophrenia. If they or their children are diagnosed in the future maybe this will give a little more understanding and they will not feel a sense of shame and disgrace as I do at times. I know I ought not to feel that way and I know it is about education but it isn't something most people look into until it affects them or theirs. I have met people who have surprised me on how much they do know and others who are professional and/or apparently well educated who have it all wrong.

Carmen and I treated ourselves to a word-processing typewriter for Christmas. We both used it mainly for letters and she used it for some of her course work. As well as being in a music club I had joined a book club and the introductory free gift was a book called 'Nil Desperandum' – Latin for all occasions. The book was another of those things I thought was sent specifically for me of all the books I got one that was about Latin. It was as if the book club were saying 'listen we know you have a problem with reading but if you can't understand what is written it may be easier for you'. The fact was it was all way above my head and as much as I would have loved to remember certain phrases I found it extremely difficult to rehearse and later recall them. Another thing about the book was it had two dust jackets and both were identical. Even though 'Nil Desperandum' translates to 'never despair' my thoughts changed to thoughts that maybe the book club was actually trying to send me round the bend and crack me up. If I never give up trying to get to the bottom of it all and get on with my life without feeling like a freak of nature I will end up being one. I cancelled my account and because the book club was affiliated to the music club I closed that account too. I had so many CD's and lots I hadn't even opened or listened to so it was probably a good thing anyway.

Dr. Breen had invited me to take part in what I assumed was a quiz for students or they could have been young psychiatrists or both, I think he referred to it as research. I entered the room and there were about 6 or 7 people and Dr. Breen who told me to answer the questions as honestly as I could do. I got the impression the others would have to guess my diagnosis. I don't remember every single question now but one of the questions was about sex being a part of me becoming ill. I told him that it was difficult to say because I was in a new relationship and we couldn't get enough of each other. I often regret not telling him that it definitely was I just didn't want to go into any of the details with him or those people in that room at that time. He could see I was being obtuse and he asked again and again I maintained that I couldn't say as we couldn't get enough of each other. I told them all about a headline I saw which read - 'Eurotrash!' All of the students were white but none were English so I assumed them to be from Europe as I am not good with accents. It wasn't a lie I had seen that headline and I mentally noted it and here I was sat in a room full of Europeans feeling like a specimen in a bottle. I recall trying to explain my problem with words both spoken and in text and about me dissecting and analysing those words. I told them also about the colours and numbers, combinations, codes and somehow being stuck inside a puzzle. Then Dr. Breen blew me away with his next question. "Tell me what sort of things the voices say". I was totally gobsmacked where on earth had that come from not my notes I hoped. "I do not hear voices I never have done my trouble is my thoughts". Dr. Breen went down in my estimation with the next thing he asked. "Ah, yes but are they loud thoughts?" I didn't know whether I was 'leaning against an open door' or whether he assumed I was that thick that I couldn't distinguish between a thought and something audible. I felt like saying are your thoughts audible but a little voice in the back of my head said, "Say yes!"

It didn't really I am just kidding but from there on in the quiz went down hill and I never did get a bloody fiver!

With help from Andy the minister from church and Margaret and a few other people I independently produced a bi-monthly Newsletter called Nil Desperandum. The help they gave wasn't so much practical help but I secured funding for type-writer ribbons and was given paper and use of photocopier etc. I put notices up in the day hospital and doctor's surgeries, libraries and the church etc. asking for letters articles or comments for inclusion. Now partly this was my own personal crusade to say look South Manchester I am a nutter but I don't feel like one. It was also partly about trying to find other people like me and users or anybody at all voicing their opinions on mental health. The first one produced had a picture on the front page of 'The Mad Hatter' from 'Alice in Wonderland' above that was the title in large font. The mad hatter in the picture was chained to a post and he was looking very miserable. There were three reasons I named it 'Nil Desperandum' the first you know about I was still not giving up my quest for answers somebody knows my situation out there. Secondly the largest font on the type writer Carmen and I had was 12pt so I cut out the title from the spare dust jacket of the book. Thirdly the title was a positive one and it all made sense. It was through the newsletter that I got to know the people who were involved with the South Manchester Users Group. The main two people of SMUG were a husband and wife team and there were some volunteers. On the advice of the people from smug I took my home address off the newsletter and the notices as they said it was 'dangerous'. Irene the nurse in charge at the Day Hospital said I could use the hospital address and so that's what I did. The newsletter got all sorts of letters and things for publication and I poached articles from other magazines or newsletters. Smug would advertise events or meetings etc. The articles or letters I got for the newsletter were mixed some from users a few from carers and of course my editorial. In issue number one. I poked a little fun at Dr. Breen and his question about 'loud thoughts' but he did tell me he read and liked that first issue.

Carmen, the children and I had started to attend church and we would try to go as often as we could. The order of service at the church on a Sunday would always be the same in that after a short time the children would go out to classes. The adults usually stayed to listen to the sermon etc. Carmen and I would take it in turns to go out with Ashley and stay with him in the class. It was usually a female member of the church who would run the class but I insisted to Carmen that one of us was always with him. This was because it had come to light that a young girl had been sexually abused by one of the church members but thankfully he had been convicted. The older three children would go into the class of an elderly lady who had been involved at the church since the 1950s. We were starting to make friends through the church and we found everybody there pleasant and friendly.

Over the next year or so the routine was the same in that I took care of the home and children whilst Carmen continued with her part-time work and college. I was still doing the newsletter and distributing it around the area and at the Day Hospital. I had stopped picking up on every headline and words etc. I was now reading without too much difficulty although occasionally I would still mentally note some headlines. I still avoided watching the telly but had started listening to radio again.

In mid 1995 I received an advertisement for the newsletter from the Schizophrenia Media Agency (SMA). They were looking for people diagnosed with schizophrenia to get involved in setting up a media agency. I contacted them and was invited to attend one of their meetings and because it was an afternoon meeting I was able to attend. Ashley was now in the reception class at school so in for the whole of the day. I didn't know what to expect as I didn't get much information on the aims of the group from the advert. It was only their second meeting so was actually the steering group of SMA and most of the people involved had been diagnosed with schizophrenia. I became a member almost straight away and got involved in what was to be the only organisation of its kind in the country. It wasn't just a case of putting ourselves forward for interviews or media appearances like I thought initially. We did all sorts of campaigning work attending seminars or annual meetings giving presentations to other groups or organisations and we also did media training. Some of the training was 'in house' and some was external it was all about getting our message across by using the media. The irony of it all was that it was parts of the media that was the problem in that their reporting on schizophrenia was not just negative but unbalanced. The language some of the newspapers used was feeding the publics fear about people diagnosed with schizophrenia. We were often 'released' from hospitals rather than discharged, we were often 'disturbed' rather than distressed and we were almost always unpredictable and dangerous. The imagery used by some of the newspapers and TV was also very negative usually the photograph being used of the person was one with mad staring eyes. Often the reason put forward for a particular act of violence was simply put down to the illness, and sometimes in simplistic terms giving people the impression that the crime was a symptom of the schizophrenia.

I learnt a lot from SMA but most importantly I met the other members of the group. There was Ollie Richards who had an encyclopaedic knowledge on almost anything relating to schizophrenia and psychiatric drugs. I met Wendy Alton a single mum and the chair of SMA she was articulate and passionate about getting a positive message across. The oldest member of the group Tom Kendall was by no means typical of any pensioner I ever knew and he again was all for the cause. Gerry McCarthy a qualified nurse was another member who believed in standing up for what we all believed in. Roger Rankin a lovely man would talk on live radio as if he was chatting to an old friend over a cup of tea in his front room. Don Royce was one of our younger members he was into the performing arts and training to become a dancer. There were other members too and every one of them different just as you would expect but all diagnosed with schizophrenia. I began to accept the fact that my diagnosis of schizophrenia may be accurate. Some of the members heard voices and some didn't but I don't recall anybody having magical powers unless you count my power to make food disappear. I never witnessed any aggression whatsoever from any of the many SMA members. As well as running workshops, training and media appearances we would have discussions on all aspects of schizophrenia. It was like a family atmosphere more than an office or meeting environment. Sometimes we would just have a sandwich and a cup of tea chatting about our kids and families not even mentioning schizophrenia. Of course I would have two sandwiches to their one and by now I was 15 stone and my family had stopped saying the extra weight suited me. SMA secured funding for a project worker and the agency was becoming known not just to the other mental health organisations but known by the media.

Members including myself were being quoted in publications as diverse as The Guardian and The Big Issue and we were being heard on both national and local radio it was all a very exciting time. The schizophrenics were talking to the public and the chattering classes by using the media. One member joked that it was a bit like the lunatics taking over the asylum now that we lived the community. We were learning how to 'sound bite' with phrases like 'scare in the community' and we want 'empathy not sympathy' and lots of others. We'd say 'well actually I have never killed anybody' and 'violence is not a symptom of schizophrenia'. There was no 'party line' or such to toe because we all had differing views with regard to medication or the care we were receiving. The main message we wanted to get across was that we are trying to get on with our lives and become a part of the communities in which we lived. We did a lot of work with Radio 4 on their various health programmes, we wrote press releases and we were being invited to give talks more often. We secured more funding to employ an overall project coordinator and were starting to produce handouts, leaflets and flyers. Sometimes the flyer or leaflet would be made to look like a newspaper with a shocking headline such as FREED TO KILL! We thought it would grab the readers' attention and it was an actual headline from one of the shit sheets. The members would each monitor a couple of newspapers each morning and if there was anything that needed to be addressed we would call a meeting. For reasons I don't have to explain actively monitoring newspapers was at times stressful for me. Meetings and training days were held regularly and we had a 24 hour telephone line with a bleeper for the media to make contact.

Now that I had an interest and home life was good I felt much better in myself it was as though I did have that job which was Anthony Scally flexible. As a family we became full members at the church and Carmen, the kids and I were all baptised. We held a party afterwards and everybody in our families came it was as if life was getting better by the day. I had gotten to know Elaine (Carmen's Mum) better and I discovered she has a wicked sense of humour that I connected with straight away. Elaine did a lot of reading and she would often give me books to read so there was always something to do whilst the family watched the telly. It was as if the work with the media agency had somehow desensitised me a little when reading headlines, leaflets, books and text in general. My routine of sleeping in the afternoon changed to one of going to bed at the same time as the kids. Dr. Breen told me I could start using the chlorpromazine tablets PRN. I was having my depot injection regularly at the depot clinic which was on the first floor of the Day Hospital. Dr. Breen made a referral to a laser clinic to have my tattoos removed and it was all done on the NHS. Anne Lorna's Mum was now living not too far from Vera, and Lorna spent a lot of time with Anne and eventually moved in with her. There's nothing wrong with that except that Vera's fears were borne out when it became apparent that Lorna wasn't going to school. Pete and Patsy were still trying for a baby and still on the IVF programme at St. Mary's Hospital. Business was going well for Pete and he had begun to talk about expanding, he already had one shop and two sign written vans. He employed three carpet fitters and was no longer having to do the actual fittings himself.

A researcher from the BBC had made contact with the media agency because a report was due out on the differences in resources available amongst the different authorities. It was about the way each authority allocated its resources more than a case of them getting different amounts. At that time Manchester didn't have a central or single mental health trust. I commented to the researcher that it wasn't until I got to South Manchester that I got a social worker. They wanted to film me getting my depot injection which was due the next day. I was a bit unsure at the time but said as long as they pixelated my arse it'll be okay. We met up the following day and I was told that the hospital would not give permission for them to enter the depot clinic. So they filmed me walking into the building and a few minutes later filmed me walking out. I didn't know whether they wanted me to rub my arse for effect or just walk out casually so I did both. I was sent back in and told to walk out again because I think I over did it when I shouted, "It's all right you're all safe now!" What went out on the six and nine o'clock BBC news was a little bit of information about the resources that some trusts used effectively etc. I was called Tony Scally 'Schizophrenia Patient' and the voiceover was the issue about not having a social worker until I moved house. When I watched it at six o'clock I thought my God you fat bastard Scally but I was pleased that there was nothing regarding violence or 'dangerous patients'. Of course by using a 'schizophrenia patient' although it wasn't said I suppose it could be construed as being inferred. It was the first time I had sat down and watched the news in several years.

Marjorie Wallace works with SANE (Schizophrenia a National Emergency) she comes from a journalism background. Her message at that time was basically there are too many people dying at the hands of people diagnosed with schizophrenia. Which is something I totally agreed with in my view one person is too many. The only thing I don't like is that it was often the illness that was put forward as to why the person had killed. There are murders happening all the time by lots of people that have never been diagnosed and don't have schizophrenia. Sometimes psychiatrists in the court setting would argue that the person was unwell when they killed. The perpetrator of the crime would then be treated in a hospital and be a patient and not sent to prison. Tom Kendall our treasurer at SMA was convinced that there were criminals who played the 'insane card'. A few months on remand to read up on things then 'I didn't know what I was doing it was the voices telling me things'. Since there wasn't a 'type 1 and type 2 schizophrenia' like in diabetes what Marjorie and the psychiatrists said affected everyone diagnosed. Sure enough as soon as somebody with schizophrenia did kill somebody else (which thankfully isn't that often) Marjorie would be on the telly. MIND the national mental health charity were different again but obviously MIND covered the whole of mental health and not just schizophrenia. They have a clearer more cogent and positive outlook. They have the right balance of the rights and feelings of individuals (service users) and the public concern for safety. I didn't know then but there had been a war of words between SANE and MIND and it started off in the London Evening Standard I think.

Four of us were sat in the SMA office watching a programme taped from the night before. It was Marjorie Wallace's 'Circles of Madness' which is what is known as an 'opinion piece.' One of the members referred to Marjorie as the Margaret Thatcher of mental health! Wendy Alton said something in German about injustice (Wendy was learning German at night school). We all agreed that when we were ill it was feelings of us and/or our families being harmed if anything and not us showing violence towards anyone else. Personally I knew no matter how ill I was I could never harm a woman or a child and would only defend myself if attacked by another male. We all thought the programme could have been so much better and positive but instead it had reinforced negative stereotypes.

I have to be careful here or I might end up being sued.

'In my opinion' it was a totally unbalanced view of people diagnosed with schizophrenia that were living in the community. It was all fairly one sided and there wasn't anything said that came across as being positive. There was no mention of people that had been diagnosed that didn't hear voices and the facts and figures (which were dubious) were about the murders or crimes. I don't recall any accurate figures about the suicides each year or of people diagnosed who had only ever had one episode of illness in their lives. It was all done very cleverly with arty imagery and haunting opera music and I am not sure but I think it got a media award a few months later.

We contacted Channel 4s 'Right to Reply' programme saying we'd like to respond to Circles of Madness. It was agreed by all of us that I would be the person who made the response if channel 4 were prepared to let us reply. They did get back in touch later that day and said they would come to Manchester the following day to film me doing my piece to camera. The way it would go out on telly was they would show a clip of what was being replied to then the piece to camera by the person replying to it. There was then a round table discussion by all those concerned which in this case was Marjorie, the presenter, me and to support me somebody named Liz from MIND.

The Manchester filming was done in one of the rooms at the building where SMA had its offices and it took almost three hours. There were several phone calls between the producer and the person in charge of the team. Basically I said what I have already told you was my opinion. At one point I stated violence wasn't a symptom of schizophrenia. The mobile phone rang again and the guy in charge answered it. "Yes just done it again but now he says violence is not a symptom". He was looking at me as he spoke to the producer, "She sez it can be an aspect". I told him hooliganism can be an aspect of football but we are not saying all football fans are hooligans are we! He nodded and repeated what I had just said into his phone and then without speaking closed the phone. He told me and the crew we had to do it again. "Sorry but you can't say that" he said. "You know this programme should be called Right to Reply errm sort of!" I said. Everybody laughed and we did it all over again but I still think the third (or was it the fourth) take would have been much better.

Ollie Richards came with me to London and we stayed at a hotel in Bayswater. At one point in the night I telephoned Carmen again to find out if everyone was okay as I hadn't stayed out overnight before. She told me everyone was fine and Chloe was looking forward to her birthday party but that two of her friends were not coming now. When I asked her why they weren't coming she told me she didn't know why just that they weren't coming. Back in my hotel room I decided that it would be a mistake to go on national TV trying to defend the actions of people who had committed murder etc. I wasn't a psychiatrist and didn't want to get embroiled in all that diminished responsibility stuff. I hardly slept at all that night thinking what it was that I was going to say. I could only speak from personal experience so that is what I decided I would do I had no script and so I thought I'd play it by ear.

The following morning after breakfast the taxi arrived to take us to the channel 4 building it was about 10am. Filming wasn't due to start until after lunch so we took up the cabbies offer of a quick tour of the sights. We were just passing the palace of Westminster when the cab driver decided to try and reinforce some stereotypes regarding racist cab drivers. "Marnchester that's full of 'Starnies' init?" We decided not to get involved in that conversation but I winked at Ollie. "I hope Willie is okay looking after my whippet and pigeons" I said. Ollie looked at me and smiled. "You remember Willie don't you Ollie, Willie Eckerslike!" For the rest of the journey Ollie and I spoke like characters from Coronation Street and by the time we reached channel 4s building we had tried to reinforce some stereotypes of our own. The taxi driver knew we were pulling his leg though because I couldn't stop laughing when Ollie said something about getting home to polish his clogs.

We were at Channel 4 for the next three hours and it was a weird day in that Marjorie and her solicitor were kept separate in the building from Ollie and me. I can only liken it to a boxing match the seconds being Ollie in my corner and the solicitor in Marjorie's corner. As nervous as I was it didn't stop me accepting and eating a tuna mayo sandwich whilst in the 'green room'. I don't know why the room where guests wait and are offered hospitality is referred to as green because quite often it's a totally different colour.

Eventually Marjorie, Liz (from MIND) and I all went into the studio and the seconds had to watch events from the monitor in the green room. The clips of film were shown and it was Marjorie who had the first word and she came out fighting. She said channel 4 had grossly misrepresented her with the compilation of clips from the Circles of Madness film. There was some discussion involving Liz, Marjorie and the presenter about figures of homicides in comparison to the figures where people who weren't ill had killed. Then Marjorie said something about me being well and her programme was about people who were unwell she said it all in a 'there there' sort of way. I told her not to patronise me this was because I had the same medical diagnosis as all of the people in her film so it affected me personally. I asked her what I tell my children when friends are kept away from birthday parties because of programmes like hers. "Do I say I am sorry darling it's because of me?" Marjorie never answered me but Liz then backed up what I was saying and there was some discussion between the two of them. It was then back to me and I said, "I have the same medical diagnosis as Peter Sutcliffe..." I paused and the light on the camera I was looking into went out and it threw me. The pause wasn't something I did purposely it was due to the tuna I had eaten 'repeating' on me and the strong taste of it in the back of my throat. I wanted to say, 'how do you think it makes me feel that people somehow assume I am just like him'. It was my 'Right to Reply' but Marjorie not only had the first word but the last word too. What she actually said with her last word I don't recall as I was still annoyed about my camera light going out. However, the presenter did say, "I don't think that's what Tony was trying to say".

The train was just pulling out of London's Euston Station when Ollie asked, "Do you remember the children's cartoon programme Captain Pugwash?" I told him that I vaguely remembered it as it was a time when I used to watch TV. He mentioned that although it was a kids cartoon there were characters with smutty names. "There was a Master Bates, a Seaman Staines and the word Pugwash is Australian slang for oral sex". I told him I didn't recall any of the characters but agreed with him that it was definitely suspect. "So you don't watch telly then?" he said. "Nope, I used to but stopped because of the adverts". He told me he didn't own a TV set and asked why I didn't just stick to the BBC as they didn't advertise. "I prefer the radio as I feel the scenery is better and besides the BBC do advertise". I explained that they advertise there own products and programmes and that advertising is something that cannot be escaped if watching sport. I told him that the BBC is not as innocent as it may seem with products 'strategically placed' in soap opera camera shots etc. I also mentioned the BBC hosting the national lottery draw and we both agreed that the lottery was a tax on the foolish. "Have you been told to avoid the TV as like in a coping strategy?" I told him I had avoided it for years even before I was ever diagnosed and if avoiding is coping then yes, but it was something I did for my own sake. "Getting back to Pugwash I believe that there are things put out to influence our thinking" said Ollie. "I agree not everything is as it seems and even before TV that was true if you think about books and by the way Pugwash was actually a BBC programme". We then spoke about Orwell of course but not just 1984, Animal Farm as well, which led us onto the topic of what is actually said or written and what it is really meant to mean. We covered lots of different books from Lewis Carroll's Alice in Wonderland right through to the writings of Nostradamus. I suggested that it was the same with some songs and even with works of art. I asked him what he knew about synchronicity and he explained that it was the theory put forward by Jung as an 'acasual connecting principle'. "Ollie it's me not your psychiatrist tell me like I am 9 years old". Ollie laughed and tried to explain it to me in a way I understood. He told me that basically it was the idea that things happen by coincidence but they seem connected. He told me everybody has experienced uncanny coincidence to some extent whether it is thinking about somebody we hadn't seen in a long time and bumping into them the same day. Or perhaps you hear a word you haven't heard before and then the following day you hear it three times. Thinking about someone and your phone rings and it is that person. Maybe going away on business and sitting next to somebody on the plane and realising that you used to sit next to them in school. Sometimes it gets even eerier in that the person only lives a few streets away and they are married to somebody else you had thought of recently. The couple have a child who sits next to your own child in class at school. "I suggest you read up on it to get Jung's actual interpretation though because there's a lot more to it". We spoke about all sorts of things but one thing he said was that he held firm beliefs that nobody can convince him aren't true and potentially can happen. "I believe that if somebody wanted to contaminate the reservoirs that serve the cities and town's water supplies then they could do, it's just a case of having enough LSD or Ricin or whatever". He went on to say, "If you think about it even if it was discovered to be contaminated what would we do for water?" We had been talking so much that I didn't realise until the train stopped we were back in Manchester. I told Ollie I would see him at the next meeting. "Right tarar then

Tony I think you did well against Marge". He put his quaraqul style hat on and walked off in the direction of his bus stop and I thought 'I wish I knew just half as much as he does'.

Apart from that first media appearance about the resources I have never watched myself on telly or listened to anything I had done on radio. Of course I would listen or watch the other members and would invariably read everything that the SMA had involvement with. The support I got from the other members and I hope the support I gave them was second to none. I got a round of applause at the SMA office a day or so after the screening of Right to Reply. I told them all to 'give over' and we got on with the meeting which was about a poster campaign we wanted to run. The response we got on the phones from other organisations and indeed journalists led me to believe that it wasn't as bad as I first thought. We also recruited more members as a result and we secured more funding for a 'peer group training' initiative. However, I knew that Right to Reply could have been so much better if I hadn't been such a greedy bastard.

Depixol is one of the older drugs that are still being used for the treatment of schizophrenia. In the years I have been on Depixol it has been called a major tranquilizer, neuroleptic and these days it is known as an antipsychotic. All drugs have side effects of some sort or other but the psychiatric drugs are notorious for particularly unpleasant ones. As well as giving me an appetite (as if I never had one before) Depixol also slows down the metabolism which is like a double negative. It's all well and good to say diet and exercise can help but being on the drug also takes away the motivation for that. It's not just a case of no inclination to cook healthy meals from scratch or to workout at a gym but having the actual energy to do it. Then there are the issues of erectile dysfunction, drug rash, Parkinsonism and others. So the debate amongst users about whether they are pro-medication, pro-choice or anti-medication etc. is an important one. It's too easy for a psychiatrist to say 'I think we need to up your meds' without them fully appreciating the physical wellbeing of the client. So that is why I agreed to be involved in a BBC Documentary programme called 'Close up North'.

The filming for the Close up North documentary took place in two locations, the meeting room at SMA's building and at our house in South Manchester. Carmen and the kids were all in agreement and supportive and the kids wanted to see themselves on the telly for sure. The producer wanted to film the SMA members having a formal meeting. We were all sat at a long oval table and there were about ten of us. Whilst the crew were setting up there was a discussion about what the caption on screen will be. We certainly didn't want the term 'schizophrenic' used. One of the crew made a comment about SMA being a baby milk and it was a shame it never spelt anything like MIND did or SANE. I pointed out that it was not always the case that it turned out for the best telling him about SMUG. He seemed to take offence at what I had said and sniggered, "But baby milk!" I suggested 'Some Mothers 'Avem and again he said it also related to baby milk and his manner suggested he was taking the Mickey out of me. I was doodling and just before we were ready to get started with the filming I had sussed it! "TEAM" I said out loud. I added the word Team to the end of the words 'Close Up North' and passed the sheet of paper to Mr. Sarcastic.

The rest of the day went fairly well we were all filmed for around five minutes of the meeting. Everybody got the chance to speak and the topic was of our personal opinions and experiences of medication. Then at our house I was interviewed in the dinning room about Clozapine (or Clozaril). It was a difficult one because in the main it is a drug that is only used where the other antipsychotic drugs had had no benefit. It has unique benefits but it also has unique risks! I was told to concentrate on the risks because somebody else would talk about the benefits in the final programme. I mentioned some of the 'less serious' side effects which were similar to those of Depixol and I mentioned others like bedwetting, drooling and dizziness. Then I mentioned the cardio vascular problems and the white blood cells issue. To finish off with I spoke about the ultimate side effect in that there had been instances of sudden death. It all became a bit repetitive because the filming was stopping and starting due to the sound engineer picking up the planes from the Airport. From the dining room we managed to film the next bit in the lounge all in one shot. Carmen and the kids were playing scrabble around a small table and I was sat in an armchair with my son asleep in my arms. In my pocket I had the letter 'S' from the scrabble board. I had told Carmen it would bring me luck as I removed it from the board whilst the crew set up. It was all I could think to say I actually took it because I knew there was the possibility of a camera shot of the board. One of the words on the board now said 'liced' instead of sliced. Call it serendipity (or more likely synchronicity if you're a psychiatrist) but I still can't think of a better word to have been there than sliced.

The word liced isn't in the dictionary but I think you know what my definition would be! Yes I know all that belonged in my kisamo box but it was a 'just in case' sort of thing.

Chapter Seven: The schizophrenia lie

It was Saturday the 5th of June 1996 when the massive bomb planted by the IRA exploded in central Manchester. Once I had established that all my loved ones were safe it was George Reynolds from ward 20 of Springfield I thought of. I wondered if he was safe and indeed if he was still in hospital being told he is paranoid and delusional. The actual explosion was less than a quarter of a mile from the SMA offices and I had to pass the area to get into SMA on the Monday. I went to collect a video cassette to use as part of a presentation I was giving at the police training college in Cheshire. Everyone in the office that morning was shocked by what had happened but for me it was more than that I was becoming worried and uneasy. I was forewarned, albeit by a patient on a psychiatric ward but all the same George Reynolds knew Manchester had become an IRA target.

Of course there are those who would say the whole of mainland Britain was always a target and again it could be put down to synchronicity. Synchronicity and not even in a rapid succession sense that can happen as there had been four years since I had met George. Without getting too complex it could also be seen as George sharing or even advancing synchronicity. We are both 'mentally ill' so why not, but this goes back to psychiatric wards and staying in our own bubble, his psychosis affecting me etc. Again I have to remind you that this is written now and with hindsight.

The agency had secured funding to employ a graphic artist to work with us on the poster campaign. Gerry McCarthy one of our members also made a personal donation of £1,000 towards the campaign. With my 'interest' in advertising I enjoyed being involved in the sessions around the messages we wanted to put out. I appeared on satellite TV with Dr. Chris Steele GP and the psychiatrist who appeared with us was a Raj Persaud look-alike whose name I forget. They were both very pleasant and it was probably one of the best things I have done on telly. It also probably had the biggest audience although in Britain it would be seen as Daytime TV. Ollie and I gave talks and did presentations at colleges, mental health groups and seminars etc. all around the country. However, we were also training some of the newer members to take up this work. Wendy Alton went into hospital as a voluntary patient at around that time. Wendy had been under a lot of stress and there were fears she was becoming ill. I went to see her on two occasions and met some of her family. I remember we had a discussion about people seeing a mental health issue and automatically assuming it meant we were below average intelligence. Wendy had some complaints about being treated like a child, oppressive nursing practice and being drugged by an ex boyfriend. It was also around that time that another member Don Royce had been sectioned. He had told the nurses I was his 'real' next of kin as I was his brother. This was because it was his Dad who had had him sectioned. The nurses were somewhat surprised when I got onto the ward because Don is Black. I tried to advocate for Don but it was difficult to ascertain from him what led to the section. The nurses refused to accept his wishes to have me as his next of kin so I wasn't told why he was brought into hospital. Don was in his room preoccupied with his New Testament and lots of newspaper clippings and he hardly spoke to me at all. I decided I would make some phone calls and get people with more experience to help him so I contacted MIND in Manchester. They called themselves Mind in Manchester and I never knew why it wasn't just Manchester Mind. I don't know whether it is something peculiar to Manchester but the university is the same, not Manchester University but University of Manchester. The next time I went to visit Don I was told nobody by that name was there and they wouldn't give me any information regarding where he might be.

The MIND Conference in Blackpool was attended by a several members from SMA we had a stand there and took it in turns to man it. Whoever wasn't taking care of the stand would attend the various workshops or presentations that were being held at the conference. The stand was just like a stall only we didn't sell anything we just had lots of information, leaflets, flyers, mission statement etc. The backdrop to the stand had black laminated boards with some of the worst headlines the newspapers had used in recent times. I was manning the stand passing out leaflets when I got into a conversation with somebody who had been diagnosed with schizophrenia. I happened to mention the analogy of thoughts as carriages on a moving train as told to me by Dr. Declan. "There's more to it than that because your filters malfunction as well" he said. "What filters?" I asked. He told me that his first psychiatrist explained in a way that suggested the brain filters out what isn't relevant to us personally. "The brain has so many filters" he said. He told me that there were filters between the eyes and the brain, the ears and the brain and even our noses. "If they are not filtering out the irrelevant stuff properly it all becomes relevant and our thoughts start to become muddled". Just then Ollie returned from one of the workshops and said, "Ah, you're talking about senses and information overload". We then got onto an American guy who once explained the mental breakdown of an individual in the same terms as computer programming. He called his theory GIGO (Garbage In Garbage Out) in other words a computer is only as good as its programming or software. To paraphrase it is when the hardware of the computer is programmed with a lot of garbage or our experiences have been shitty ones eventually all that shit comes back out. In other words part of our brain is just like the brain of a computer, the central processing unit (CPU). Another part of our brain is where everything is stored just like a computer has a hard drive and then there is memory etc. The software installed onto the hard drive (in our brain) is our life experiences and events in our lives. The breakdown or malfunction happens when the CPU (in another part of our brain) tries to process the faulty data. GIGO is an actual computer term and does mean exactly the same thing. However, most of what is written about it would suggest that computers 'unlike humans' process every bit of information not knowing it's flawed or irrelevant. I didn't attend any of the workshops or talks etc. at the MIND conference. I did have the most informative and interesting of conversations though and mainly with people who had mental health issues.

Carmen and I decided we were going to tie the knot and the date was set for March 22nd 1997 just six months away. Anne was also going to be married, both her and Lorna were going to relocate to North Wales with her new fiancée and his children. Brian's Mother had made contact through one of Carmen's family so Carmen and the children met up with her. It wasn't too long after, that Brian himself made contact and started to take the children out each Sunday. I was pleased for the kids but Carmen was still very bitter. Carmen, Ashley and I continued to go to church although there were some Sundays when we never went mainly because I would not feel up to it. Church was becoming a problem for me there was so much symbolism and ritual involved. Now you'd be surprised how much symbolism or even 'visual aids' are used in services, it isn't just the cross and the chalice. As for rituals again I was surprised that there was more than just the taking part in communion. Andy Knight informed the congregation one Sunday that he and his wife were leaving the area because he was taking up another post. Carmen had passed her exams in typing and computer studies etc. and she got some regular shifts at a local home for the elderly. I continued to take care of the home and kids and I would always try to fit the SMA work in around my domestic commitments. My Sister Karla had separated from Wayne her husband and I hadn't seen her in over a year. I was losing Dr. Breen as my psychiatrist as he was focusing on research and only working in the mother and baby unit of the psychiatric hospital. My tattoos were completely gone and unless you knew, it was as if I had never had them. Dr. Breen before leaving had taken me off the chlorpromazine completely because there were fears I was developing tardive dyskinesia. Tardive dyskinesia is a medical condition involving the involuntary movement of lips, tongue, mouth and facial muscles. It is brought on by long term use of 'dopamine antagonists' (Drugs that are used to block dopamine such as Chlorpromazine). It can also effect other extremities and once established can be irreversible. It was around this time that I received a signature only 'application' for a credit card in the post. I hadn't applied but apparently there was an American Express card with my name on it waiting to be despatched. It wasn't a gold card but green and I was unsure of the amount of credit. The paperwork was limited to just the one page for the signature. When it arrived I told myself I was going to use it sensibly and the limit turned out to be £15,000! The new minister at church was the Revd. Sarah Fellows and she and I hit it off straight away. We had many conversations on lots of topics and surprisingly very few about religion. My new psychiatrist was to be a Dr. Harry Docket and I always refer to him as Harry but I never did in his presence.

"I am not a service user I don't like the term user, I am not a client I am a mental health survivor or simply a survivor". I looked across to the table opposite and at the person I had just overheard. He had a goatee beard and had a small silver cross dangling from his ear. Beneath his black leather Jacket he was wearing a 'loony tunes' T shirt featuring Daffy Duck and Porky Pig. I told myself I must try and have a chat with that guy after lunch. Tom Kendall and I were at a hotel in Scarborough for two days where I had been booked to give a presentation about the work of SMA. There must have been 150 people and the majority of them service oops 'survivors'. Thinking about what goatee beardy man had said I thought about the importance of language again. It was actually something I was going to talk about in the presentation too. Of course I knew that there were some survivors/users who will never accept the term 'mental health problems' it had to be mental health issues. Political correctness was coming into its own at around this time, 'issues' because there were some who didn't see their 'illness' as a problem although both words can be interchangeable. So I began to wonder why survivor instead of user and thought perhaps they didn't 'use' any psychiatric services or social services etc. Perhaps it was because they had come through their 'emotional experiences' and out the other side intact so to speak. I had mental images of people clinging to the wreckage in the wide open sea. Maybe it's because they haven't become a suicide statistic or it could be all of those things. Then there was the phrase used by everybody about overcoming tribulation 'you'll be alright you're a survivor'. "You not hungry then?" asked Tom. "No such thing Tom it's like saying I don't have a hole in my arse". There may have been 150 or so people but I bet there weren't many who didn't hear Tom's howls of laughter. The event had been organised by UKAN (United Kingdom Advocacy Network) who were based in Yorkshire. They offered an advocacy service, support, encouragement and befriending mainly. Like most organisations in mental health though they are also a campaigning group. I never did get to speak to the guy with the goatee but I saw another man whose dress sense suggested he may have been diagnosed with schizophrenia. I remembered from my research in 1992 that there was sometimes an 'outlandish' or 'peculiar' way of dressing amongst some schizophrenia patients. Now I don't recall it being seen as a symptom but seen more as an eccentricity or oddity. Ollie Richards as far as I recall was our only member who dressed in this way but to a lesser degree than this guy. "Hi I am Tony Scally" I said as I offered him a cigarette. "I know who you are" he said accepting the fag. "So when you gonna be on with Raj?" I laughed and told him at SMA we call Raj Persaud rent-a-psychiatrist and I lit my fag and gave him the lighter. "In the survivor movement you are known as rent-a-schizophrenic or professional schizophrenic" he said as he gave the lighter back. What he had just said hurt me I was sat there in the hotel lobby feeling wounded and somewhat offended. If I could have walked out and got a train home without losing face I would have done it that instant. I am not really the thick skinned sort of person, and as he hadn't said it with venom but matter-of-factly I assumed it to be true. It was only half an hour earlier I was beginning to get excited about mental health again and considering putting more time in at SMA. I knew now though I was going to drop out of mental health campaigning altogether and try and get on with my life.

The following day I did do the presentation and it went down like a lead balloon. I caught Tom unprepared when I asked him to give me some support and I was actually heckled by one guy in the room. I was using a flip chart to try and emphasise what is actually said or seen and what is actually inferred. The problem was it was advertising I was using as my example of how the media has its own agenda. As I sat down my face as red as a beetroot even Tom said, "You're good at bullshitting that's for sure". If only they had caught some of the other presentations I had given where I had been confident and on the ball. Tom apologised for not coming up with a sound bite when I had asked and I told him it didn't matter. It really didn't matter I was going to be married and spend more time with my family I had done my bit it was now time to get on with life.

Dr. Harry Dockett was a GP before becoming a psychiatrist, a Martin Bell sort of character in that he only ever dressed in a khaki jacket and trousers. He seemed to know all about my involvement with SMA so I assumed he must have spoken with Margaret Warburton. Although it was only the second time I had seen Harry I negotiated a change of medication from the depot to an oral one. I told him I wanted to go onto a different 'typical drug' called Sulperide and I had read up on it in the BNF. I chose Sulperide because it was a case of the side effects being less in particularly with regard to gaining weight and erectile dysfunction. "Sulperide is a respectable drug" he said. "Well I wouldn't go that far and is there such a thing of any psychiatric drug?" I asked. "I mean it is well thought of or highly regarded" said Harry. I told him I would get back to him and let him know about that one. Now I don't doubt that some psychiatrists may have experimented with taking drugs recreationally or possibly just at university or med school. It's something a lot of professionals as students have done and indeed some are still doing. So psychiatrists may have actually experienced paranoia and/or visual hallucinations and maybe even auditory ones too. It could even be seen as personal research I suppose. Being paranoid about not getting a dissertation or thesis done or hallucinating that a piece of furniture is made out of elastic is quite different though. I don't want to generalise but your average psychiatrist when at university etc. has not had a life that can compare with many of his or her future patient's lives. There again I am not saying that everyone diagnosed with schizophrenia has had a traumatic childhood or adolescence either. From the people I have spoken to over the years it does seem to feature though in a lot of cases. Tripping cannot really equate to mania or psychosis unless the person dabbling in the drug has underlying issues. In saying all of that though I have heard of instances of people having one 'bad trip' and it leading to a diagnosis of schizophrenia. In a way it's virtuous of the student psychiatrist to try to get an idea of what it may be like. It would be a good defence too especially if they are caught with LSD or cannabis etc. in their possession. I am not saying that all psychiatrists have experimented with hallucinogenic drugs or marijuana and amphetamines etc. I am saying even those that may have done still have no idea how it really feels to experience mental illness. Obviously apart from LSD (LSD has been used in the treatment of some psychiatric disorders including Schizophrenia), the drugs used to treat schizophrenia are never experimented with in the same way. So there can only be an understanding even more tenuous of what it actually feels like to be on an antipsychotic drug and on it long term. This is why I feel that it is the better psychiatrist that will listen to what the patient has to say with regard to the meds. Harry in my opinion was one of the better psychiatrists. To be honest I hadn't met any of the worst kind of 'trickcyclists' but I knew they were out there.

I was sat in one of the cells at Grey Mare Lane Police station in East Manchester. I was not going to be interviewed until the morning because I had nominated my fiancée to sit in on the interview. I knew I had the right to a solicitor but I also knew that because of the schizophrenia I had the right to nominate a 'responsible adult'. Usually it's the person responsible for the care of the person arrested like a social worker. Margaret Warburton was probably in China half way down the Yangtze River on a cruise boat when I needed her that November evening. I phoned Carmen and told her I had been arrested and I asked if she could come to the station in the morning once the kids were in school. I started to recall how I came to be here whilst looking at my sore and red knuckles and the blood on my tracksuit bottoms. I knew I could probably end up being sent to prison but I just didn't care. I didn't sleep that night I couldn't it was as though I was in shock and I was very tearful, the only person on my mind was Lorna.

It was three weeks after returning from the UKAN conference in Scarborough and two weeks after my outpatient appointment with Harry. I was due to visit Vera and I didn't want to be out late as I was feeling a little tired. I didn't fancy the journey across town on the bus so asked Carmen if she would drop me off. It was about 5pm so to get back at a reasonable hour I said that if she dropped me off I would make my own way home on the bus. We had a row about it because she had refused saying, "You've got a free bus pass so I am not using 'my car' like a taxi". My point in the argument was that I thought it was a family car so was actually our car. I also didn't understand why she would see me as being nothing more than some freeloading passenger looking for a lift. I did go on the bus in the end and I had told her I would stay over and probably for a few days. I felt we needed some time apart especially in light of the argument we had just had. It meant letting her down with the children, so she was going to have to phone in work with an excuse.

I arrived at Vera's House at about 7pm and she saw the small suitcase I was carrying. "What's happened now?" she asked. "We've had a row I am staying here a few days if that's alright". Vera told me that of course it was okay and said, "You're supposed to be getting married in a few months". I told her that although I loved Carmen I was beginning to see a side to her that I just did not like. "It's like that for everyone I bet she feels the same about you at times" Vera said. I thought about what she had said and there was so much I did like about Carmen. Vera was absolutely right about the best of couples getting on each others nerves now and then. I started to feel like a bit of a pig in letting Carmen down with the kids so she was unable do her shift. "Yeah you're right I'll go home in the morning and make it up with her" I said. "So how's everyone Mam?" She told me Lorna now had a tutor who taught her from home. Lorna was now living with her Mum and her Mum's new husband in North Wales. Whilst in Manchester prior to them leaving she had missed a lot of schooling. I say missed schooling it was by choice just how she came to be given the right to choose I don't know. Lorna had just turned 14 and apart from the first year of high school she hadn't been regularly since primary school. I was worried because I could see a pattern developing in that it was similar to my own schooldays or non-schooldays. Vera told me Pete was doing alright and she filled me in on what my older two half brothers and their families were up to. I told her it was Karla that I hadn't seen in ages and asked about her. Vera told me she had separated from Wayne but I already knew about that as Pete had told me. I asked Vera why they had actually separated and she told me I should ask Karla that question and not her. "I am supposed to be meeting Karla and Simon for a drink in half an hour" she said. Simon was Karla's lodger and I cannot be 100 percent sure but as far as I knew it was all strictly above board and platonic. "Right I'll come with you but I don't want to have too many as I am on new meds".

Vera went and sat with Karla and Simon and I said I would get the drinks in. Karla was drunk when we arrived so I only got her half when I got the round of drinks. Simon didn't drink alcohol so the conversation with the barmaid was one of me trying to ascertain whether a can of coke was cheaper than draught coke. I hadn't been in a pub at night in quite some time not being a drinker as such. I have never been a big drinker and almost always it's to celebrate an occasion, at a party or times like these so I am probably a 'moderate social drinker'. The pub seemed a bit lively with a lot of laughter and I got a sense of people being happy it was that time of year. Christmas was on its way and the songs being played on the juke box as well as the decorations were all festive.

"Well I think Ant should know" said Simon as I approached the table. I put the drinks down on the table and sat down next to Vera. "I should know what?" I asked. I looked at Karla who was sat facing me she was obviously too drunk to string together even a sentence. "Know what" I asked again, this time I looked at Simon. "It's Wayne" he said looking at Karla. She made no response and just then Vera burst out crying. "It's about our Lorna isn't it" she said between sobs. I looked at Simon again and again he looked at Karla and she looked at me but was having difficulty keeping her eyes open. Vera still crying put her hands to her ears saying, "I don't want to know I don't want to know!" With hindsight I feel this was a case of her having an idea of what had been going on but not wanting it to be confirmed. "Well I bloody want to know!" I said to Simon. "Stop fucking around, tell me!" Simon didn't drink or smoke but he was a stoner all the same in that he only ever ate the stuff. He wasn't very bright and with a limited vocabulary, he had lodged with Karla and Wayne and when they separated decided to stay at Karla's. "He's been shagging your daughter man!" I didn't finish my drink I stood and as I left the pub I heard Vera screech, "He's going to kill him".

About 10 minutes later I was knocking on the door of the house where Wayne Dawson lived. The light was on in the downstairs front room. A curly haired young woman opened the door and I walked straight in and as I passed her she fled through the same door. He was sat bare-chested in an armchair in the front room and as I entered he stood. I head butted him and he fell back into the chair and I knew I had just broken his nose. He tried to stand again and this time I punched him below his chin and fired a volley of punches about his stomach. Between each blow I told him he was a dirty bastard paedophile and he was going to be prosecuted and sent to prison. He did fight back but his attempts were feeble and it only added to the amount of times I hit him again. It ended up me sat on his chest just punching him about the head and face. Now Dawson was lean but quite tall and always gave out that he was a rough and tumble hard bastard frightened of nothing. He was one of those people who talked a good fight usually against two or three and he always came off the better etc. just a gobshite basically. He started shouting KATY! STEVIE! at the top of his voice. Then I heard there was a little girl crying upstairs, it was my niece, I never hit him again after that. "Clean your self up and I'll see to Katy and Steven". I lit a cig and my hands were trembling so badly I thought I was going to drop it. Then my nephew entered the front room he had come down from the bedroom. "Steven go back upstairs and see to your sister" I told him. He was crying and said, "Uncle Anthony I will if you don't hit my Dad again". Now

Dawson knew me well enough to know that once I was aware there were kids in the house he wasn't going to be hit again. "He won't Stevie, will you Ant?" I called him pathetic for screaming in order to wake the kids. I should have known though that Karla and Dawson were 'sharing' the 3 kids so that they'd each get social security entitlement and rent paid etc. "The police are on the way you know, Abigail will have phoned them" Dawson said. I told him I was going nowhere and when they do arrive he will confess what he'd done to my daughter. "Karla can't see to the kids she's pissed so when your girlfriend shows up sort it out because I am making sure you get arrested too". The kids were still crying upstairs so I went up and he followed me and as I entered my niece's bedroom I heard the police radios on the stairs behind him. Dawson said, "It's not me it's him". I turned and the policeman that passed Dawson in the doorway said, "You've obviously assaulted this man so I am arresting you, now don't make matters worse, come on". He had the cuffs ready and I held up my hands for him to put them on me. He snapped them onto my wrists and I did drop the fag as the right hand cuff caught the bone of that wrist. I stepped on the fag telling him he wouldn't get them any tighter without drawing blood. Another policeman right behind him told Dawson the ambulance was on its way and used his radio to request that a female officer attend the scene. The kids had calmed down a little and Dawson entered the room from the doorway and sat down at the end of his daughter's bed. "He is a paedophile and the filthy bastard has been sexually abusing my daughter" I said pointing down at him with both cuffed hands. It was as if they didn't care or they hadn't heard me. As I was led out of the room I said, "You're going to prison Dawson". Both policemen tried to lead me down the stairs each gripping me around my arms just above my elbows. "Listen these stairs are not wide enough I am not going to do anything or run off". One of them let go and the other led me down and outside then into the back of a police van. As we left the street I could hear the sirens from the ambulance as it approached and passed us on the road. I manoeuvred my hands in order to look at my watch but I couldn't see the time as the glass covering its face was stained with Dawson's blood.

I was kicking myself for not realising the younger two kids were still living with him. I wondered why Karla chose to have my twelve year old niece Carol live with her and leave the younger kids with him. I deduced it must be because of her age in that Karla must know he's into kids, but surely not his own children! Katy was four years old and Steven was eight at the time when Karla separated from Dawson.

I told them at the police station about my diagnosis and that I wanted my fiancé present at the interview as my 'responsible adult'. "Don't talk shite you can have a solicitor and that's it". I told them that they should already know all this if they knew PACE (Police and Criminal Evidence act 1984). PACE was something I knew about from the training event I was involved with at the police college. I also confirmed that of course I wanted a solicitor present as well. "Schizophrenia eh lucky you're not on a murder charge then aren't you?" said one of them. I told him it was never my intention and he said it was only because I didn't have a gun or a knife at the time. I was fingerprinted, photographed and I gave a DNA sample I also handed over my shoelaces when they asked for them. As well as the mug shot the backs of both my hands were photographed too. I got to make my calls at 11pm and afterwards I was taken back to the holding cell. I asked about a cup of tea and my medication. "Fuck off nutter you think this is the fuckin' Ritz?" I said, "fair enough" and asked for water with my meds. "Got to have the pills checked out by the police doctor first" he said. "I am not particularly bothered about you calling me a nutter but do you have kids of your own?" He told me that if I was allowed to go around taking the law into my own hands we'd all be living in the jungle. "You're right, I know you're right, I didn't think, all I thought about was my little girl". The same policeman came back five minutes later with one of my Sulperide pills and a plastic mug and it did actually contain tea. He gave me a light for my cig and said, "Try and get some sleep nothin's gonna happen now till mornin".

The next morning I didn't deny anything I had done and I told the police everything with as much detail as they asked for. I had already related the details and sequence of events to the solicitor earlier. Carmen being there was just for support more than anything but also I didn't want to relate what had happened more times than was necessary. The interview was all tape recorded and I read and signed a written statement. During the interview I was shown photographs of Dawson's face his ribs, chest and stomach etc. just why I was shown them I don't know. "Do you expect me to feel sorry for him because I do not" I said. The solicitor had already told me earlier that I may be remanded and not get bail. Thankfully though I was granted bail on the condition that I didn't go anywhere near Dawson or try to contact him.

Leaving the station in the car with Carmen I noticed a Vodaphone advertisement on a huge billboard and it would have been hard not to notice it. It shouldn't have affected me as it did because I hadn't missed a single dose of the Sulperide. Whilst I was on the Depixol although I saw the ads it wasn't such a problem. Adverts have changed over the years in that most have taglines and this particular Vodaphone tagline was – 'How are you?' and Vodaphone has had a few, another example being – 'Tell us what you think'. All very clever and my personal opinion was too bloody clever, this wasn't concern for me or for anybody else for that matter. I thought perhaps they were trying to get information, in other words they were 'on a fishing trip'. Even if it were just a case of 'please choose us as your network' in theory they can collect information about people. Who we call, what we say, text messages, our location and who calls us etc. it was all very 'big brother'.

I wasn't aware of course but I was right back where I was in 1991 I was ill again.

I didn't have schizophrenia at all I had been diagnosed with it so that I could be controlled with drugs and not be aware of what is really going on. Everything that had been put down to illness in 91 was all part of what was happening now it had been happening all along. I had believed the 'you're not well you have schizophrenia' lie, and they got me hook line and sinker. There are lots of other companies with taglines of course and all of them became relevant over that Christmas period. I use Vodaphone as my example here but there are lots of them and each has a shared agenda. By January the kisamo box exploded and the contents which I had added to over the past 6 years were all intermingled with everything else. It then became a case of it all being around my life personally, not just me but my kids and my family. I had been given the diagnosis so that they can set me up, the trouble was 'they' could have been some of the people I once had in the kisamo box.

As you have probably guessed I didn't put Dawson in the kisamo box. There was no such box now I had lost insight completely. In January 1997 I stopped taking the meds I needed to keep my wits about me!

Chapter Eight: Going to America

In February I attended the magistrates' court in
Manchester, I pleaded guilty and I was bailed to appear
at the crown courts for sentencing. The stipendiary
magistrate had asked for reports to be done by the
probation service and the social services and for them to
be ready for the judge at the crown court. I was totally
unwell standing there in the dock in my new navy blue
wedding suit wearing a bright orange tie. At one point I
told my own solicitor in open court that my medical
diagnosis has nothing to do with what I did and being a
father had everything to do with it. The Magistrate told
me off but in a kindly way I felt. "Mister Scally you
leave the defence to your legal team please and besides
this isn't the time or place anymore". The magistrate
then had a few whispered words with his clerk of court.
"Dawson has been charged now your Worship" said my
solicitor as the clerk sat back down. "You know that is
immaterial and it's highly unfair, it's out of my hands
now" said the magistrate.

Margaret came to see me that same week and Margaret
being Margaret told me in an upbeat way that I ought not
to worry. Of course I didn't tell her about the adverts,
the things people were saying, the real thing that is going
on and I never told her that I was only pretending to take
the meds. I didn't tell her that I was worried and not for
the obvious reason that I was facing a minimum 2 year
prison sentence. I didn't say that I had been listening and
digesting every possible news bulletin that I could and
that it was news that was worrying me. Nor did I tell her
that my last credit card statement told me I had notched
up over £2,000 with my erratic spending. I had overdone
it spoiling the kids and family members over Christmas
and buying them all 'special gifts'. Each present
symbolised companies, shops, or brands that I felt could

be relied upon or trusted should anything happen to me. I didn't tell her that the 'Express' (Daily Express) headline I saw recently led me to believe that the 'Express' (American Express) would be my lifeline. Just as I hadn't told Harry any of those things and it wasn't that I saw either of them as being 'involved' in any way. Just like me they had both been led to believe I had schizophrenia so they were doing their best to care for me and indeed it was their job to do so. It wasn't a case of me believing that there was no such thing as schizophrenia (although there is a school of thought that says there isn't), just a case of me being wrongly diagnosed. Diagnosed to take away my credibility, diagnosed to be set up, I see the bigger picture and no government wants that.

In March the school opposite our house took its five foot perimeter fence down and over a two day period a twelve foot one was put up in its place. It had been the year before that Horrett Campbell had gone into a local school in the Blacknall area of Wolverhampton. He was armed with a machete and during the children's teddy bears picnic he attacked and injured three young children and four adults. In March 1997 he was sentenced and it was news again and more details were released such as him seeing the children as 'little devils' and him suffering severe schizophrenia. He was found guilty and sent to a secure mental hospital for an indefinite period. I took the fence thing personally without considering that a lot of schools were concentrating more on security these days. It was also the previous year that a lone gunman went on a shooting spree in Dunblane Scotland. I remember at that time being furious that one of the first people asked to comment was Marjorie Wallace. It was at a time when the motive was still unclear and the news media had to rationalise it by saying he was mentally ill. They couldn't say Thomas Hamilton was a bad bastard bearing a grudge, and even when that came to light there were still those that said he must have had underlying mental health problems. Call it paranoia and not necessarily my paranoia but I felt that the school fence was excessively high and it was looking more like a prison than a school.

Once we had found out about Lorna being abused Carmen had given up her work and became my official full-time carer. The Rev. Sarah Fellows visited me one afternoon and asked, "Have you seen the journalist sniffing around outside the church?" Apparently he was looking for a story because the ex church member who abused the young girl had been released from prison. Now the young girl who had been sexually abused happened to be related to somebody I knew and got on well with. Nothing odd about that because I had met the relative through the church, what did affect my thinking though was that, that person had enduring mental health issues. I needed time and space to think, I was due to be married in two weeks and I was unsure whether there was anything I could do in the meantime to 'put everything right'. There were too many distractions at home I was beginning to get upset and tearful for 'no apparent reason' at times during the day. I was also very protective of the children, being very anxious if they were outside of the house playing on their own. I told Carmen I was going to spend a few days away and on my own. "I need to sort my head out" I said. I made her promise not to let the kids out of her sight and I let her think it was Vera I was going to stay with.

Later that evening I phoned Carmen from the Portland Thistle Hotel in central Manchester. "Are you sure you want us to get married because you do know I may end up in prison?" Carmen told me that she definitely did want us to marry and not to worry about the court thing as we'd cross that bridge when we came to it. I wasn't worried about the prison thing particularly but I had to tell her that that was the reason we ought to think about not marrying. I couldn't tell her what I felt was really going on, that I was in danger again and that it may affect her and the kids. The solicitor told me worse case scenario may mean going to jail but it wouldn't be a typical prison sentence. "You'll be looked after and treated as if you were royalty" he told me. Carmen told me that Ashley and the other children wanted me to come home and that she and the kids would always be there for me. "I may be taking a flight to Dulles International later" I told her. "What are you talking about and where are you now?" I told her where I was and that I need to sort everything out and that Dulles is in Washington in America. "Tony have you got your meds with you?" she asked. "Yes I have and please don't worry because I will be home in a day or so and will phone again before then".

I had booked and paid for the flight by telephone from the hotel room and I used the American Express card to pay. My ticket was waiting for me at the Virgin Atlantic desk in the departure lounge of Manchester Airport. To me it seemed that the world had so many problems, problems that seemed not to concern others. Whether it was radio or TV news, with each new bulletin there was yet another catastrophe about to happen, and it was all linked. I was fearful for everyone and could not understand why others seemed oblivious to the whole state of affairs. The name of the credit card itself 'American Express' led me to believe I needed to get to the USA and as soon as possible. I don't know why but I assumed that Clinton was expecting me and not for one moment did I think that any door would not be opened for me. The song 'Change the World' by Eric Clapton and some other songs I had heard at that time also made me think it was something I just had to do. Now I didn't know that Bill Clinton was busy 'splashing out on a new dress' for Monica Lewinsky at around that time. It was some British election news in the end, as well as my conversation with Carmen that made me decide not to take that flight.

I only spent an afternoon and one night at the Portland and the following morning Carmen came in the car to take me home. The car was parked on double yellows whilst I paid the hotel bill and collected some orange shirts that I had in my room. "Tony why do you have so many orange shirts?" asked Carmen. "I bought them yesterday and I really like the colour". I put the shirts onto the back seat of the car and returned to the hotel reception where I handed over the American Express card. "That'll do nicely" said the young woman with a giggle. The room cost me around £80 and I had made four phone calls; two to Carmen, one to Virgin Atlantic and I spoke to Vodaphone! The conversation with Vodaphone was a brief one in that I told them, "I am fine thank you for asking, oh and by the way the future is bright the future is orange". The operative asked me whether I had the right number stating, "This isn't Orange we are better than Orange". I told her that of course she was bound to say that and I ended the call thinking my exact location was being sought by their satellites.

The preparations for our wedding were well underway, Elaine had made the dress for Carmen and bridesmaid dresses for the girls. Lorna, Chloe and Amanda were all going to be bridesmaids and all of them were excited and looking forward to the big day. Lorna was still in North Wales with her Mum but was going to stay with Vera for the weekend of the wedding. We decided that we would marry at the registry office in Manchester which happened to be on the same site as the Magistrates and Crown courts. Carmen's Dad Barry was going to give her away at the ceremony and Carmen's older Brother Keith had arrived from Jamaica especially to attend the wedding. Elaine and Barry had divorced when Carmen and her siblings were quite young but Carmen had maintained contact with her Dad. Barry had remarried and has another daughter by that marriage, Carmen's half sister Gillian. Gillian and some other relatives on her Dad's side of the family were all invited to attend the ceremony and the reception event afterwards. I invited all of my friends from the SMA and my family including my Aunts and Uncles who I hadn't seen since Pete and Patsy's wedding. A friend of Elaine and her family had agreed to take the photographs and Carmen's sister's boyfriend had already made the cake. Everything was set for Saturday 22nd of March which was about a week away.

I had a routine outpatient's appointment with Harry four days before the wedding and Carmen came along with me. It was a nice day weather wise and walking across to the entrance of the hospital I spotted a lone magpie. I have never been superstitious but on this occasion I scanned the whole of the area that was in view praying that I spotted another one. I was paranoid out of my skull noticing everything and everything being connected and relevant, and I had been that way for the past few weeks. I don't know why but I felt special or important though and quite invincible. The paedophiles, druggies, bent policemen and government flunkies were not going to get the better of me. It was different than my 'first episode' experience of 1991, in that I wasn't afraid, but everything else was exactly the same. The colours, adverts, news bulletins, registration numbers, signs and all the symbolism were back and I was trapped in the puzzle again. "How are you sleeping and how is your appetite?" asked Harry. It's a question I have been asked so many times over the years that I imagine it being drummed into the psychiatrists during their training. I imagine them all having to recite it over and over and their teachers telling them, "Now you all know that this is the key that will show the symptoms". Some people have the romantic notion that psychiatrists have unlimited time, small caseloads and a comfortable 'couch' for their patients. It is the common mistake of confusing a psychiatrist with a psychologist or what are known in America as 'therapists'. A psychologist doesn't prescribe drugs and the therapy is a 'talk therapy' whereas a psychiatrist treats symptoms of illnesses with drugs. I think the confusion has arisen because in the states in certain circumstances there is an overlapping of 'talking' and the prescribing of medication. It is a Hollywood image and indeed it is probably the rich and famous who have such clinicians to talk to and get their Prozac from. Amongst that group of the Hollywood actors and the rich and famous etc. there is even a certain degree of esteem and it is seen as trendy to have such a therapist. In Britain and away from Harley Street things couldn't be any more different though. So I fully understand that it isn't always easy for the NHS psychiatrist to come across as taking the holistic approach. "My appetite and sleeping are both fine" I lied. "It's just that you are getting married in a few days and with what has happened with your daughter... I don't want you to become ill again". There was no couch and as is usually the case I was sat furthest from the door with psychiatrist nearest to it. "You and I both know something is going on, even the birds outside know it" I told him. "Like I said you don't want to be unwell and frightened again at this time in your life". I stood up and said, "I am a Scally and I know I am not bullet-proof but I am frightened of nobody, I have the balls of an elephant!" I dropped my trousers and then my orange boxer shorts and Carmen started laughing. "Perhaps this is a good time to reinstate the depot injection" Harry said. Now I thought he meant because I was stood there with my pants around my ankles not because I chose to show him my bollocks. I told him I would take on anybody man to man but that I cannot fight who I couldn't see. "Things are being said through other people and those people are like a conduit being used to crack me up". I pulled my pants up and although it was incongruous behaviour I never apologised. I just didn't care, everybody was going along with life as normal whereas I knew so much. If only they knew and could see the whole thing and the bigger picture, all I wanted was for somebody to say 'yes you are right'. I was a maverick and on my own I couldn't talk to people about what was going on just in case they were part of it. I needed for somebody else to let me know that they knew and I had to decide if those who didn't know really didn't know. So people were either involved, in the dark or pretending to be in the dark because they were involved. Between Carmen and Harry I was persuaded to go back onto the depot, Harry told me that it was only to stabilise my thoughts. "You have a copy of the BNF let's just get you through the next couple of weeks". I trusted Harry and Carmen and I don't know why but I thought Harry knew about what was going on globally and locally. He knew I was caught up in it all and I knew he wanted me to get through it safely. It was also a case of me thinking that the wedding and being a married man is what 'they' didn't want and potentially it was my 'winning move'. I had the depot injection of Depixol. As the needle went into my arse I said, "You know this means I won't have a decent honeymoon". I was referring to the erection problems and what it would mean going back on it. I forget the dose I was given but it made no difference as I lost the plot a few days later.

I had arranged to meet my sister Karla in central Manchester I told her that I wanted her and the children at my wedding and that I would buy the clothing. So now she had no excuse not to come to the wedding because I did feel that it was an excuse them all having nothing to wear. The wedding had been on the cards long enough for her to sort something out if she really wanted to attend. Karla had all of the children living with her at this time and although Dawson had been charged he was on bail and still at large. I bought the outfits for them all from Debenhams and as we were leaving the store Karla told me something that still makes me sick now.

Over the years some people have had a direct impact on my mental health some of them unwittingly and not realising, and there are some who have set out to make me ill. It sounds like an ambiguous and a negative statement that somebody would purposely set out to crack me up but I believe it to be true. In Karla's case and on this occasion I am sure it was thoughtlessness and her not fully appreciating my fragile state of mind. I have said before that people can't know what other people are thinking and unlike a physical illness there are no outward signs of being unwell. As you already know I myself when unwell quite often dismiss the whole schizophrenia thing and put it down to being controlled.

"Wayne has been phoning my house upsetting the kids, saying really horrible sexual stuff" said Karla. We were walking away from Debenhams and along Market Street and I remember there was a busker and he was playing the violin, badly. "Saying stuff about girls having two holes and them liking cocks up their arse" she said. In my mind I was transported back to the age of 13 and it was as if it was only then at that time that I fully appreciated the true extent of what Lorna must be going through. The thoughts of guilt and shame and at that age not being able to fully understand what or why it was happening. It seemed like a million things flashed through my mind all at once including the comment by the obnoxious service user from the day hospital. He made the comment about having sex with a 13 year old virgin so he must have known this was going to happen there was no other reason why he would say such a thing. "I should have fucking killed your husband, tell the bloody police!" I said to Karla. I was that angry as I spoke that when I did there was breathlessness and I only just managed to complete the sentence. It wasn't just anger though I wanted to collapse onto my knees and cry my bloody eyes out. I quickly told her I had to go and that I would see her and the kids on Saturday at the registry office. I was heading back down Market Street and passed an electrical store and there was an 'Orange' advert in the window. A few minutes later I ran back along the street and caught up with Karla again. "Here, screen your calls and if he is stupid enough give the tapes to the police". I handed her the answering machine I had bought from the electrical shop and I told her it was just a temporary measure until she gets her number changed.

I didn't fall to my knees but I did sob all the way home on the bus. I didn't care that people were looking at me and I didn't answer the one person who asked what was wrong. As I have said Lorna was still in Wales and although we had spoken on the phone I wasn't able to bring myself to discuss with her what had happened to her.

That is still the case to this day, after all it isn't until now and me writing this book that anybody knew of my own experience with Burnett.

The morning after meeting up with Karla I was woken by Carmen, "Tony what's happened in the lounge there are books and CD's all over the place and bits of paper everywhere?" I hadn't had much sleep in fact I was getting into bed just as Carmen was waking up so it couldn't have been much more than 15 minutes. "Yes it was me I was trying to work things out" I told her. "The satellite doesn't work either why is that?" I admitted to her that I had put the receiver into a sink full of water so that it wouldn't ever work. "Well you better get up and sort the lounge out and you can phone Sky to get it repaired, I am going to phone Margaret". Suddenly it was like Ping! I was wide awake again so I got up out of bed I had things I needed to do. I had to get to the shops to buy some bottled water.

What had happened the previous night and in the early hours of the morning was a sequence of events that started with a child's drawing. It was at about 11.30pm, Carmen and the children were sleeping and I wasn't tired so I decided I would tidy up around the house. In the dining room whilst sorting out a pile of papers on the table I became aware that it was actually drawings and paintings that had been done by Ashley and Jerome. They had been brought home from school and upon further inspection I realised it was all of their schoolwork from the previous year. I immediately phoned the police and they arrived about 30 minutes later. I was waiting at the front gate when the squad car pulled up and there were two policemen both in full uniform. "Mister Scally?" asked the older policeman. I nodded, and asked if they wouldn't mind turning their radios down as my children were sleeping. One of them was a white middle-aged stocky officer and the other a slim Asian policeman who was about my age. It was the older policeman that did all of the talking and they both sat down on the couch in the living room. The coffee table in front of them had a cardboard folder containing all of my 'evidence' in the order that I wanted to show it to them. "Now before I start I want you to know that I have alleged mental health issues but this has nothing to do with that". I opened the folder and showed them a photograph of Jerome it was taken in a classroom and he was scowling and not at all happy. As I passed it to the older officer I said, "You see thing is I think there is child abuse going on, possibly a paedophile ring". I went on to say that if we could find out who took that photo we'd know more. Then I showed them both a painting done by Ashley, "Can you see it, he's crying out and in pain" I said. "Mister Scally if you think we can start an investigation because of some children's drawings you must be mad". I told him that me being mad was debatable and asked if they couldn't just make discrete enquiries. "On Monday you phoned us from your neighbour's house stating your life was in danger and your phone was tapped, now who is your doctor?" I told them that my life was in danger but that I wasn't scared anymore and now they are getting at me through my kids. "Is your GP on-call at night?" I knew I was wasting my time and assumed them both to be bent coppers and the look in the eyes of the younger one made me think he definitely knew something. "Who is it?" the older one asked. "Who is what?" I replied. "Your GP!" I told him I had tablets in the house and I didn't need a GP or a psychiatrist. "Just give me a name, take your tablets and if we get anymore calls from you I will know who your doctor is". I told him the GP's name and he wrote it in his notebook and as he did he spoke the name slowly. He spoke it in a way that seemed exaggerated and he had split the surname into two words. "Doctor….Water…House, right take the pills, your kids are safe and so are you". With that they both left, I didn't take any pills of course, I couldn't I needed to stay alert. I spent the next 4 hours or so on one of those mad missions. I unscrewed plug sockets and light fittings looking for listening devices, I re-examined the evidence of the paintings etc. I looked everywhere for the answer of how I could take on and beat these despicable criminals who had government backing. I started thinking that the Labour Leader who had died in 1994 (John Smith) had been killed. I couldn't think of anywhere else in his home that he could have had a heart attack and end up with water in his lungs other than in the bath. (Of course I didn't know he had water in his lungs it was an assumption and I also assumed there had been a cover-up). Shit! That's it, they are going to try and 'doctor the water of my house'. The copper isn't bent he is helping me 'Doctor Water House' it was a clue! I even remembered that on the train coming back from London Ollie Richards had mentioned contaminated water as well. I thought I would be able to use the Express card to buy bottled water from now on. I switched off the supply at the stopcock but not before I short-circuited the satellite box with a sink full of what I assumed to be poisoned water. I was dying for a cup of tea as well, and then I spotted a bottle of coke on the kitchen counter and took a slug from the bottle. Yuck! The cola was warm and flat, I looked in the fridge and we had plenty of semi-skimmed. I poured half a pint of the milk into a pint glass and topped it up with the flat coke and I decided I had just invented 'moke'. I sat on the bottom step of the stairs in the hallway drinking the moke which actually tasted divine and I can only describe it as a liquid mars bar. I lit a fag and as I smoked it I was feeling proud of myself, the bastards, I have foiled them!

I said right at the beginning of this book it hasn't been easy to write and it hasn't and not just for the very obvious reasons. It has to be an honest account but there are things I just cannot relate such as other peoples real names. Dr. Waterhouse is a health professional so it doesn't matter so much that I mention him as being a part of my muddled thinking. The names of some of the other people who I know or who I have come into contact with, just like any other word, phrase or piece of text are all open to 'manipulation' by me. It wasn't always the case as it was the Dr. Waterhouse name that started that ball rolling so to speak. Nor can I relate all of the things that are currently detached within my head in the box I have called kisamo. It isn't about upsetting people however much they may have upset me at the time. I don't want to go into too much detail of my love life (or non-sex life) or Carmen's physical needs, and I don't want to sling mud at either of our families. This book is about schizophrenia and I think what I have already written should tell you by now that of course, real life runs alongside things imagined, assumed and any sort of symptom.

Carmen did phone Margaret that morning and it must have been Margaret who contacted Harry and Dr. Waterhouse. Between Carmen and the three of them I was sectioned on the 21st of March the eve of what should have been my wedding day. It was mid afternoon by the time I got to Withington Hospital and I hadn't slept in 36 hours. There was no force used and I didn't need to be restrained I went along voluntarily and I was as high as a kite. It wasn't a drug high it was all natural that is unless the properties of the moke had chemically reacted. I was back in that 'zone', I was invincible, clever, on top of the world, I was excited, elated and I wasn't a bit frightened. I actually thought that the hospital was the forum in which I could get to the bottom of everything I was Manchester's very own James Bond. The copper had told me my kids were safe and he 'told' me that it was the water supply that they may try to doctor and I was going to ensure that everyone knew.

Chapter Nine: Somebody's watching

Harry disappeared when we arrived at the hospital and I presumed he was organising a place for me on a ward. Margaret and I were in a waiting area and I asked her whether she was going to be okay and would she be safe. Margaret assured me that she was perfectly alright and to stop worrying about everyone else because everybody was safe. I started to think about Carmen and our planned wedding and I felt it was all my fault that now it wasn't going to happen. I only changed the meds in the first place because I became aware that Carmen seemed worried. Now I didn't for one minute ever think her worrying or her moodiness had anything to do with concern for my mental health. Carmen told me on more than one occasion that she couldn't see me as being ill and she only saw me as being a bit eccentric at times. That for me was absolutely the best thing she could have said, however it's then that other things come into play. My sleeping and lack of enthusiasm or inclination to always be bright-eyed and bushytailed would mean I was lazy or that I didn't care about life. So I put the moods and her worried looks down to our upcoming wedding and that she may be having second thoughts. There were also the conversations we had that usually started with me apologising and ended with her saying that sex wasn't the 'be all and end all'. As I thought about it though I was glad I had changed the meds because if I hadn't I would still be in the dark about the important thing that was really going on. I was happy that I was no longer being kept in a chemical state of naivety or unawareness and I thought that there must be others who could see it all too. I began to wonder whether there really is such a thing as schizophrenia and perhaps there are others diagnosed who are being kept under control. I liked Harry but there was no way I was going to go back onto the Depixol or any other drug for that matter.

A bed had been found for me on wards P-5 and P-6, yes it was just the one bed but the ward was known as 5 and 6 because it was actually two wards that were joined in the middle. Once I got onto the ward I was shown the room in which I would be sleeping and Margaret left saying that she would see me after the weekend. The bed in the room hadn't been made up yet and the fitted wardrobe was empty. Somebody had scraped into the varnish of the wardrobe door and there was a crudely drawn crocodile with the word 'reptile' below it.

The TV was on in the lounge area of the ward and I am not sure whether it was the lounge of ward 5 or 6 but it was the side where my room was. There was a male patient not much older than me sat watching the telly and there was another man in his 40s stood by one of the windows. I lit a cig and sat down and the programme on the box was a quiz programme. I remember there were three contestants and the questions were multiple choice answers A, B or C. I watched and listened and I soon became aware that there was a sequence to the answers and it went C, B, A and then A again. It meant there was always a B after the C and then after the B two A's, then a C again. I started to give my answers out loud and sometimes was firing off the answer before the question had even finished. This went on for a few minutes and the two patients were by now paying full attention as my answers were parroted on telly. The patient who was seated got up at one point and looked behind the telly and from the telly he walked to where the aerial wire went into a socket on the wall. The older patient who had now come across from the window was stood next to where I was sat. He said, "Pull it out Sam". The other patient pulled the aerial wire from the socket and obviously the picture on the TV turned to one that was distorted. There was a slight hissing sound but I could still clearly hear the questions and so could both of the patients. I could see that the older patient who was hovering over me was becoming agitated so I shut up. Then he picked up an ashtray from the table in front of me and emptied the contents onto the floor. He then threw the empty tin ashtray towards the back of the lounge and at the same time the other patient switched off the telly. I was still sitting and the younger one walked toward me stopping directly in front of me with only a small table between us. The older one was still standing to the side of me and it was he who said, "He's one of Hitler's boys Sam he's a bastard German". I felt a bit threatened and as there were two of them I thought about shouting for help. I stood up and as if by magic a male nurse arrived into the lounge area, the older patient returned to the window and the other one sat back down. Margaret had told me that she would let Carmen know which ward I was on so I decided to wait for Carmen in my room.

I don't know how long I had been sleeping on top of the unmade bed but it was still daylight outside when I woke. It could have been for a few minutes or even for a few hours but when I did wake it felt like I had slept a while. I got up and noticed that the door to the wardrobe had been opened so I looked in it and it was still empty but on the shelf there were two blue tablets. I looked at the tablets and I knew that they were both 10mg Valium tablets I didn't know who had put them there or why. I thought perhaps it was a clue so I played about with the letters of the word 'Valium' and then 'Diazepam' and how they may be connected to the crocodile on the wardrobe door. I sat there with the two 'mothers little helpers' in my hand sorely tempted to just swallow them but I never. I took the tablets directly to the ward office and demanded to know why they had been put in my room. I was told that nobody knew anything about it and it was suggested that it could have been one of the other patients. I didn't believe a word of it but the Valium I felt was definitely put there by an ally, Harry perhaps. I didn't take the tablets because I didn't feel I needed to and I never wanted to miss something that may be important. Since waking up though the elation and feelings of excitement had gone I wasn't frightened but there was a definite feeling of apprehension. Nobody told me but I had decided that there were many other people who knew what was going on nationally and globally. Again I wasn't told but I decided Margaret and Harry both knew about it and they both knew that there was something being done to address the situation. I wasn't a danger to myself or others I was a 'loose cannon' so to speak and may mess everything up for those who can address the situation. Nobody told me any of that I deduced it because of the tablets that had been left for me to find and take. I went back into the lounge area and the telly was on again and it was a news report all about smoking and passive smoking. There was a female patient sitting down watching the telly and her packet of cigarettes were next to the ashtray on the table in front of her. I noticed they were a brand called 'Royals' and I started to recall the incident earlier with the patient who threw the ashtray. I was certain it was all connected but what on earth are they trying to tell me and not just the patients but the BBC too. I made my way to the ward exit and was halfway down the stairs and almost outside when a male nurse stopped me. He put his hand on my shoulder as if making a citizen's arrest and he quoted some nurses code about him being able to section me. Now I thought I was already sectioned so didn't quite understand what he was talking about but I did agree to go back with him onto the ward. I turned the telly off and sat down in the now deserted lounge and I was hoping that Carmen would hurry up. "Anthony I am Ernie I would like you to come downstairs with me to a much quieter ward". I looked up and there were three male nurses and one of them was a massive guy who looked like any typical nightclub bouncer. The other two were of average build and Ernie the one who had spoken had a striking resemblance to Andy Knight the ex minister from church. I knew that this wasn't really a request to go with them more a case of 'come with us and come quietly'. The 'bouncer' tried to grab my arm and I said, "I will come with you to the other ward but do not touch me because I don't need help in getting there". As the four of us passed the ward office to leave the ward I heard a female nurse speaking on the phone, "Yes Anthony Scally is now on his way down to P-1".

I don't recall how many wards there were at Withington Hospital on the psychiatric side but all of the wards had numbers and began with the letter P. I assumed that the P stood for 'psychiatric', these days though the wards in a lot of psychiatric hospitals have names rather than numbers. Withington Hospital was actually the former Chorlton Workhouse so it is highly probable that it had been treating the mentally ill for many years. In most towns and cities there is usually one or more of the psychiatric facilities that has a reputation for not being a very nice place. There were stories (and jokes) about the patients of course, but there were also stories of maltreatment of the patients by other patients and/or by the nursing staff. In Manchester top of the list was Prestwich Hospital, everybody knew it or knew of it and everybody had a different story to tell. The two factions for the different aspects of story were either 'ordinary' people telling tales of mad people or former patients relating their experiences of the hospital. When I was sectioned for that first episode of illness in 1991 I had heard of Springfield Hospital myself and it was in the way of it being all about the 'nutters'. Since moving to south Manchester and being a service user at Withington Hospital though, it wasn't the hospital that I had heard of in the other way at all, it was just the one ward and that ward was P-1.

Ernie pressed the buzzer to the electronic door of ward P-1 and we were buzzed in, the two other nurses didn't enter the ward and left as soon as we entered. As soon as we were on the ward Ernie went into the ward office which was close to the electronic door. "Hang on there for a minute" he said. I stood waiting outside the office when another patient came and stood next to me. The patient told me that he was the 'one and only Henry Vance'. "Roy Orbison had a relative called Billy and I think you are Billy, Billy Orbison, get it, Billy!" he said. Although I didn't know him he looked and acted as though he was just on the borderline between being 'a bit merry' and being sober. After he spoke it was as if he was a comedian who was telling a gag and waiting in anticipation for laughter. He had a mischievous smirk on his face and there was a definite twinkle in his eye. A male nurse further along the corridor asked him whether everything was alright and if he was okay. "Sound as a brush me, sound, just that I initially thought he was Billy". Henry winked at me and went along the corridor and onto the main part of the Ward. Ernie came out of the office and told me he would show me around the ward once we had had a chat. I was still thinking about the Billy thing when another patient started shouting. "That fucking Ernie doesn't believe in God watch him mate". I did turn as Ernie opened the door to a room further along the corridor but there were several male patients in a seating area so I had no way of knowing who had shouted it. Once inside the room I asked him what all that was about him not believing in God, and how did the person know that he didn't. "He asked me and I told him because I don't believe in it, none of it, when we die we are worm food there is nothing after that" he said. I told him that although I didn't worship that often on Sundays I was actually a member of a church. "Yes but do you believe it all?" I had to concede that when I did go to church I only went to 'edge my bets' and at the same time see if anything persuaded me. I said that as yet I hadn't decided if I did believe it all or not and that it was really difficult for me to do so. Difficult because I sometimes avoided the sermons, services and readings in the same way I avoided the other things that I felt affected my thinking. I found Ernie easy to talk to but it was weird with him looking so much like Andy Knight and us having this conversation. "You're dead right you know because I don't think religion is helpful especially where schizophrenia is concerned" he said. He went on to explain that whatever the religion was when people hear voices they assume it must come from their God and they look for answers in their particular Holy Book. "They assume the book is written by their God and not by mortal men of many years ago" he said. He also stated that it was common knowledge that the Christian Bible for one is open to interpretation or translation and that is why we have ministers. "If it was straightforward we wouldn't need vicars' etcetera and there wouldn't be different versions of it either". I told him that I personally didn't hear voices but that I have had trouble with words and reading. "You don't know what is happening to you and you are looking for answers but you are lucky not to hear voices" Ernie said. I told him that I didn't believe I truly had schizophrenia and whether religion is helpful or not I thought that the people who do believe in a God are not bad people. "I am not saying that they are but we can't generalise can we, think of some catholic priests with their alter boys and think of the Wars all stemming from religion". He then said that the irony of it all was that if Jesus Christ was to be on earth today he would be sectioned. "Why would he, he was never a danger to himself or others?" I said. Ernie told me that perhaps it would be the case that others were a danger to Jesus and he went on to say, "And again it's ironic but probably some of the preachers of today would pose a risk and therefore the way he acts makes him a danger to himself". I said, "So is that why I have been sectioned then?" He looked at me and smiled "I don't want you to think like that and I can see I am going to have to watch you mister Scally". I told him that I didn't want him putting something in his notes about me thinking I was Jesus because that wasn't what I meant. Ernie laughed and told me that nursing notes were not half as bad as some people said they were. He told me that although it was never proven David Koresh of the Waco cult fame definitely had schizophrenia. "He was so intelligent, articulate and convincing that his followers the Davidians were just blown away by him... and literally too" he said with a laugh. I thought about what Ernie was saying and was beginning to be sorry I had even mentioned him not believing in God. Ernie told me that he firmly believed in the fine line between genius and madness but as an intelligent person he could not believe in God. I told him that there are lots of highly intelligent people who do and that whether Jesus was the son of God or not he only taught all good things. "No offence but I'd rather not discuss this anymore right now" I said. "Fair enough, your fiancé is bringing you a change of clothes at seven and you can use the office phone if you want her to bring anything else". I told Ernie I needed a shower as another patient initially thought I was Billy Orbison and I also said that I wanted to appeal against the section. He looked at me quizzically and told me that he had never heard of Billy Orbison and I told him that nor had I but that 'initially' it is B O! Ernie laughed again and he told me that the ward clerk will get the paperwork together about the section after the weekend. "There's something wrong with both of the showers so you may be better off having a bath". Ernie gave me a tour of the ward and that was the last time I ever saw him.

He was quite right there was something wrong with the showers in both of the bathrooms because I had tried using them. The problem was getting the temperature right as it was either too hot or too cold and just when I thought I had cracked it, it ran stone cold again. I didn't take the advice of having a bath and in the end I decided to have a strip wash using one of the washbasins. I was sat on the edge of my bed in the male dormitory dressed in just my boxer shorts and I was thinking of the titles of Roy Orbison songs. It wasn't too long before Carmen arrived with sandwiches, toiletries, cigarettes, loose change for the payphone and some clean clothes etc. It was as if I hadn't seen her in years she looked so beautiful and everything about her was vivacious, fresh and so perfect. I got an immediate erection so she pulled the curtain around the bed. We kissed and I manoeuvred her hand toward Mr Happy and two minutes later it was all over. "You wouldn't believe I have had two cold showers would you?" She asked me why I had been thinking about it at a time like this so I explained it wasn't until I saw her that I did think about it. I told her it was a joke about the showers because they were faulty and most of the time I had been thinking about what the heck was going on. "Nothing is going on you're not well Tony and don't worry about the wedding because everybody understands". I told Carmen I intended to appeal and that we would eventually be married and I assured her that we would be even happier than before. "I believe you but that means you are going to have to accept the medication" I also told her I am not the only one who knows what is going on with the media who I referred to as the ministry of truth. "You really need to accept the medication Tony". I felt a lot better after Carmen's visit she seemed upbeat and positive and didn't seem to be too put out by the cancellation of our wedding. This could have been due to her mother Elaine saying that she wasn't happy about her ex husbands daughter Gillian being invited to the wedding. So now Carmen had the time to try and diplomatically sort it out amongst her family so that her mother did actually attend. I could have been wrong but as I say she didn't seem to be overly concerned by it all.

At that time an appeal against a section 2 could be heard by an appeal tribunal anytime after the first 7 days and almost always within 10 to 14 days. However, it was variable as it could depend on public holidays and weekends etc. So in effect, of the 28 days it was possible to be lawfully kept in a hospital for half of that time before it is decided if the section 2 is even justified. Just like any legal appeal or hearing there are notes to be prepared and read and of course the appellant has the right to have legal representation. In my case and on this occasion it was going to be three days before the process would begin and my intentions were officially known. Whilst thinking about it all I had eaten all of the sandwiches and was ready for a cigarette. I decided that I would bite the bullet and sit in the communal area designated for smoking, the lounge.

The lounge was a large open space with no doors and it was impossible to enter or leave the ward without using the long corridor which made up part of the lounge. There were chairs around the edges of the two end walls and more chairs all along the large metal framed floor to ceiling windows. The windows made up the longest edge of the lounge and looked out onto the enclosed garden that was also part of P-1. In a way it was like a huge glass wall and there were heavy curtains hanging at either end as if they were in the corners of the room. Beyond the garden and one story higher I could see the lit up windows of the ward opposite and there was somebody stood at one of the windows. There were three male patients all seated in the lounge of P-1 and one female patient who seemed to be pacing one small area of the floor. Henry Vance was sat facing the windows and next to his chair was a bright pinkish fluorescent or day-glow traffic cone, and printed on the cone in black was the word 'SECURITY'.

I entered the lounge and sat down between two of the patients with my back to the 'glass wall' and I was directly across from Henry. I removed and lit a cigarette from a full packet of 20 and almost immediately the female patient asked me for a cigarette. I am not tight-fisted by any means and don't like to see other smokers without a cigarette. So that is why when I had phoned Carmen I asked her to bring some rolling tobacco and cigarette papers so that I would be prepared. I offered to make her a roll-up cigarette and she looked at the 20 filter cigarettes in my hand. "Sorry these are all I have got and I don't want to run out of any". I rolled the cigarette gave it to her and she put it in her mouth and I gave her a light. "You Crafty Bastard, I fucking like it though" Henry said laughing. Cigarettes in my personal opinion are an integral part of ward life and I learnt it very quickly back in 1991. Previous experience had taught me that it can be a costly business and a little bit like feeding a wild animal in that they keep coming back for more. Smoking is an addiction so if there is a supply available people without any will ask those who have some. I personally go without before asking people I don't know, and it can be very difficult at times to do that. Then there are those patients who 'ask' for a cigarette in a threatening or demanding way, firstly to get the cig but also to establish whether you are frightened. I have seen patients hand over cigarettes because they are frightened of refusing and sometimes their families are funding half of the wards habit. Of Course there are plenty who may only ask occasionally and always return the cig or cigs as and when they get their own. Just as you may expect not all psychiatric patients smoke but again I have known non smokers ask family to bring in cigarettes too. They then offer them out in a way of forming 'friendships' or more likely they are looking to feel safer. There are some patients though who just don't have visitors and don't get any or enough of their own cigarettes. There is also the situation where patients who don't get many cigarettes will request that the nursing staff 'mind' their cigs for them. Most of what I am talking about refers to patients encountering first episodes of illness and are themselves afraid of other mentally ill people. There are some 'difficult' patients though who never get to see more than one cigarette at a time as the staff will always look after their supply for them. Their own cigarettes are then used as a reward for good or appropriate behaviour. It is known as 'a token economy' and is an approach I saw used at Springfield hospital and I didn't like it. With schizophrenia it is widely believed that it does work and that it works better with the negative symptoms. So patients who have difficulty with social interactions or taking care of themselves may appear to benefit in the short term. The problem with it for me was when the same approach was used for patients experiencing hallucinations or delusions and other positive symptoms. If you let somebody have their cigarette as a reward it stands to reason that by not giving it you are in effect punishing the person by actually withholding what is theirs to start with. Now this is not to be confused with rationing or making the cigarettes last for the patient or the cigarettes being looked after for patients who give them all away. Sometimes even if that is the reason for the cigarettes being kept by staff they may still be used as tokens for those patients. The tokens should really be all about reinforcement but I have seen it used purely as withholding for punishment and the punishments far outweighing any of the rewards. The patient becoming more distressed the longer the punishment or withholding of the token goes on and then that distress is seen as poor behaviour. Whilst at Springfield I witnessed patients having to be forcibly medicated as a direct result of the way the 'token economy' was implemented. Also whilst I was in Springfield I gave away so many of my own cigs that I had no option other than to learn quickly or quit. As you can imagine going cold turkey at a time in your life when there are so many other things going on just never happens. There are people who may disagree but for me a token economy using cigarette tokens at a stressful time isn't right. If it was a classroom and the tokens were tubes of Smarties it would be entirely different again. Nicotine though and the addiction to it coupled with the proven fact that people who do smoke can get a sense of calm tells me it is totally wrong. In a way it is just like bribery but the bribe has actually been stolen from the person you are offering it back to. Not only that but they want it so badly and they want it because it is theirs and the longer it is kept from them the more stressful it is. You would think the staff would go out of their way to maintain a calm and peaceful ward but like I say there is the punishment aspect. People who are unwell can make accusations, derogatory remarks and insults against members of their own families. So the nursing staff are by no means excused from any of that indeed they are more often than not likely to be on the receiving end of it. Some of those same staff may then decide to punish, but it is the loop in which the patient is punished and the patient may then react against the punisher. Sometimes the way around that one is to punish with medication the medication wears off and the cigarette tokens start all over again. I don't call it care it's all about making people acquiescently subservient or docile and not always because of what they may have done just what they may have said.

I don't want to come across as generalising but it does happen and I have witnessed it happening at Springfield. I use the term nursing staff to include qualified and non-qualified people working on a ward. I concentrated on my own experience of care at Springfield and as you have read it was on the whole fairly good. There were patients though who weren't so fortunate for whatever reason and I questioned the whole thing once I was discharged.

Henry said, "Laura you can get ciggies for your side effects love, you just need the right doctor, Doctor Lambert or maybe Doctor Butler". Laura put the last vestige of the roll-up into an ashtray and left the lounge and I could hear her laughing as she went. "She gets a hundred a week every week and she doesn't get to see or smoke half of them" said the older patient sitting to the right of me. I thought to myself 'so that shit still goes on does it, if I get time off the ward I shall buy hundreds of cigarettes courtesy of American Express'.

I decided I liked Henry and I thought perhaps this was someone who had a way of thinking that was just like my own. I had once heard of a patient and she gave all the psychiatrists who she had dealings with appropriate names that were linked to how they prescribed. Dr. Hal O Peridol, Dr. Thora Zine, Dr. Stella Zine (possibly related to Thora), Dr. Sara Quel and other names that I don't remember. I was thinking about sharing this with

Henry and the other two. Then the older patient who must have been in his 50s complained about the TV not working. "That bitch on P-10 hasn't got a telly either, always staring at us down here in the fish tank" Henry said as he pointed to the upper ward through the window behind me. I didn't say so but I was glad that the telly wasn't on because I didn't want to know about anything in the wider world. The patient sat to my left who was aged about 40ish then spoke for the first time, "Everything on this ward is fucked up even us". I couldn't resist making the comment that even the showers had bipolar disorder. There was just a titter from Henry and then suddenly all three of them started to laugh and the laughter rose to a crescendo and a male nurse appeared on the scene. Henry pointed at me and said, "Billy reckons" he paused and started to laugh again, "that the showers have got fuckin' manic depression". The nurse smiled and said, "What on earth goes through your minds at all". Henry said, "Well you had to be there". The nurse looked puzzled, "Be where?" Henry started laughing again, "In the fuckin' shower". I was pleased that I had broken the ice with three of the patients but the 'security cone' and the person watching from ward P-10 made me stop and think. I was thinking lots of things but mainly I thought I must stay in my own bubble and get out of here so I can marry the woman that I love.

The Saturday that was supposed to have been my wedding day I got several calls to the ward and the staff allowed me to take the calls in the office. Tom Kendall phoned to say he was on his way in to see me and I took that call on a grey telephone, and on the same phone a little later I spoke with Vera. My brother Pete phoned to say he would visit me mid-week and that call came in on a brown telephone and so did another call minutes later which was from Carmen. I tried not to look too much into it but I would be lying if I said it didn't worry me and occupy my thoughts all of that day. As I have already said as well as the government, the advertising, national and global events my thinking was all connected to my personal life. I was paranoid and although I managed to separate some aspects or at least worry less about them paranoia can not just be switched off. The feeling of me being important was mixed in with it all and it was in a 'show off' way too. I was important because I was 'a nobody' from a council estate in Manchester ready to take on and expose it all and aren't I so very clever. The problem was I had no insight whatsoever and it was as if there had never been a kisamo box. It meant there were child abusers, disgruntled ex husbands and crabs, there were partners who had cheated and they were possibly cheating again. There were incidences of things that had been said and done by me, about me or to me. There were life events and the feeling of wanting to protect my kids and all of it was no longer separate but part of that paranoia. It was all so very complicated and there were so many strands to my thinking. To try and concentrate on one strand I just could not do because that one strand 'wanted' to interweave with all the others, it was impossible. Harry wants me on the medication so I don't come to any harm he surely knows I am not mad. Carmen knows nothing of the bigger thing she only has an insular stance on most things so perhaps it is the person she is seeing who wants me on medication. Oh yes I believed she was seeing somebody forget about illness and think about how Carmen and I met because it was always in my mind. He wants me on medication because like me he cannot bear to think of anybody making love to her better than he can. Perhaps I am caught up in some sort of love triangle maybe he is a married man or maybe he is using Carmen to get to and abuse my kids and step-kids. It could be the same man who gave her the crabs or it could be just another affair and maybe that is why Carmen isn't bothered by the cancellation of our wedding. Thoughts like all of these and others as I say were on my mind not just since the phone calls on the ward but since I was arrested for assaulting Dawson. Carmen maintained that she did actually want us to marry though and that is why I didn't make any direct accusation of infidelity. Could it be that she is using me like some sort of pawn, using me in a way of marrying me to spite or enrage her latest fling or indeed her long-term affair? Not only was I totally in love with Carmen but walking away from her meant walking away from another of my own children. If you knew Ashley and the way he and I were together and how happy he was with his mum, me and our family unit you'd know that that was never an option for me. There was also the whole thing about him being of mixed race amongst Carmen's family. A family where two family members had shown 'anti-white feelings' towards me and others in the family had definite issues around interracial relationships. Then there were my own brothers and my sister and the things that had been said. Members of both of our families were just more strands and they really belonged in the kisamo box, but like everyone and everything else they were running loose within my head. Also running loose were policemen, doctors, solicitors, Christians, atheists, gangsters and water contaminators. There were so many strands to the way I was thinking all entangled and jumbled up. There was definite worry but also a certain amount of audacity or a feeling of invincibility 'alright you bastards I'll take you all on'. Irish terrorists were in there too not just running loose but they were all of them entangled or acquainted with the other strands, put simply I had a head full of chaos.

There are instances of people on psychiatric wards either sectioned or as voluntary patients that are only there because of very real fear (no I mean warranted fear). Yes they may be paranoid and yes they may be reacting oddly as a result of it but a psychiatric ward is probably the safest place to be in the community. It is far safer than a prison cell but not as safe as being in a different community many miles away from the first one. Inner city psychiatric wards deal with all kinds of psychiatric illnesses but they also deal with drug induced psychosis or just people who are part of the whole drug culture. Manchester like many other places has its families and individuals who don't really need to live off anybody else's reputation. Dealers, gangsters, doormen, racketeers, 'businessmen' or thugs, you can call them what you like. I am certainly not going to name any names here but they are people who have influence. They can usually get things done either by themselves (acting together) or more likely somebody does it for them. That may include getting somebody to malinger his way onto a ward to deal with Joe Bloggs or 'get into' the other patients heads and they will deal with him. Joe Bloggs may consider himself streetwise or think he has that inner strength to get through the ordeal. He may not care that his peers say that 'Joe has gone under' or it may be that he really has 'gone under'. Going under is a term used by some drug users and it simply means that the drugs have gotten the better of you. Maybe there isn't even a malingering aspect to sorting Joe out, 'that mad bastard with the psychiatric problem that knows a friend of a friend' will deal with it for the 'baddies'. When I say deal with it, it could be physical violence or it could just be about getting Joe 'psychiatrised'. The 'battleground' or arena is the psychiatric ward and rightly or wrongly there may be other patients who genuinely fear these families too. Poor Joe Bloggs may end up diagnosed and labelled indefinitely and it is highly likely he's more scared of the family, families or individual than before. Joe may also end up on medication for a long time too and I believe this in itself can bring on real mental illness. I am not saying either that Joe Bloggs may not have had real mental health issues from the start it's this whole thing of seeing the bigger picture. Seeing the person not just Joe the 'symptom' walking around nervously but thinking about Joe himself not just what may be going on in Joe's frontal lobe. Of course medicos can only treat in a medical way but if they truly believe they are helping the patient they cannot insist it's all delusional. This in itself can add to Joe's distress and may have him think that even the doctors and nurses have been 'got at'. It can give the baddies even more influence or at least the impression that they have more. If Joe is lucky enough to be given a social worker then that person needs to be listened to as well. I also disagree that somebody has to be diagnosed in order to be treated, especially for a first episode of illness. Depending on their motive one thing is for sure the baddies will either get their money, get to screw Joe's wife, get him to smuggle/deal drugs or get him to commit other crimes for them or something else. These families or individuals who usually work with each other always get things done by a third party and the third party does it to gain favour. I am not saying either that Joe is an upstanding citizen himself because I know of a Joe who isn't but he most definitely isn't mad either. Perhaps Joe has given evidence against someone or it has come to light he is a police informer whatever it is the baddies get their reputations by sorting the Joe's of this world out. It's a street reputation and not something you are likely to hear on the news but word does get around. What is worrying though is that out there in Granada land there may be mental health 'professionals' and/or agency nurses who know of their reputations too.

So when I talk of safety or security on a psychiatric ward, patients or nursing staff being threatening or not taking the chance of being in a bath full of water you now know why. I don't use street drugs or mix in those circles and haven't since the 80s so it shouldn't really concern me, but it does concern me because I know it happens. It may not happen that often but it happens far too often to be swept under the psychiatric carpet. There is also the fact that I didn't know who it was that Carmen may be seeing behind my back. It is a fact that I didn't know and not a fact that she was seeing anybody I need to add.

All of the tea cups on ward P-1 seemed to be plastic yellow ones all except one which was a plastic green one. I had tended to use the green one since arriving but I had asked Vera to try and find me an orange plastic mug. There were more of the patients sitting around that morning some waiting for visitors and some with visitors. There were empty chairs but it was difficult with the way that everybody was spaced around not to sit next to somebody. I eventually sat next to a young man in his late teens or possibly early 20s whose name was Alan. "What have you brought me?" he said as he rummaged through a carrier bag. His mother had brought him crisps, a litre of coke and 40 cigarettes. He ate two packets of crisps in what seemed like half a minute with no qualms about the noises he made. "Where's mi dad?" he demanded to know from his mother. "Alan you know we don't visit you at the same time" she said calmly. Just then two young blonde haired twin girls aged about five or six entered the lounge each of them holding the hand of an adult who I presumed was their dad. "Awwe just look at them two" said Alan's mum. The girls and their dad went directly toward a young woman in her early 30s who I assumed was the twin's mother and his wife or partner. I also assumed that at the very least the patient hadn't eaten much in a long time and the expression skin and bone just about summed up her appearance. Alan's mum got into a conversation with another female visitor who was sat with Henry and she told her that she was Alan's main carer. "He stays at his dad's now and then as well" she said. Alan started guzzling the coke from the bottle and the gasses in the drink made him cough repeatedly. "He's so intelligent you should have seen some of his school reports and all the certificates he has, it's such a terrible illness" said Alan's mum. Alan lit and started to smoke one of his cigarettes and he did so in the same fashion as he had eaten the crisps. He was taking long hard puffs and breathing in the smoke noisily. "When's mi dad coming?" he said as he exhaled some smoke. "It'll probably be this afternoon love I don't know" she said. Henry announced to everybody in the lounge that he really really loved his wife Louise. Louise smiled and told Alan's mum that they weren't together anymore. "You still love me though don't you" Henry said. The twins, their mother and their father made their way to a smaller non-smoking room which was also where the payphone was. Laura came through into the lounge and asked Alan for a cigarette and she thanked him when he gave her two. Laura sat down in the empty chair that still had the security cone next to it and smoked one of her cigs. At one point she burst out laughing for no apparent reason, the laughter turned to a whimper and then into sobs and then there were tears. A male nurse came into the lounge and Laura stood up dropped the dog-end onto the floor she then stood on it and wiped her eyes. The nurse walked towards her and she purposely sidestepped him and made her way back towards her room looking back at him as she left. "Bloody hell if looks could kill" said Henry to the nurse. "I don't know why because we usually get on" the nurse said. I crossed the room and sat in the chair where Laura had sat and whilst sitting there I wondered about what it means. Was it that whoever sits here offers security to everyone else or was it that it was the most secure place to sit. I looked out of the window and up towards ward P-10. Blimey! Either I had just hallucinated or there was a glint that could have been from binocular lenses and it came from the person who was stood at the window up there.

I realised during my time on P-1 that anybody who claimed to be 'anti-psychiatry' really didn't know what they were talking about. To me it was an education and the realisation of just how necessary psychiatry is and how much that it has to deal with. Still though, there are people who I met at the time and have since who just didn't and don't fit into psychiatry's neat and tidy boxes.

During the 10 days or so that I was on the ward I got visits from my family, and from Carmen and some of her family. I was also visited by the Rev Sarah Fellows and by SMA friends. Dr. Dockett and a junior doctor who worked with him agreed to my compromise of me having the orange largactil and only that. I didn't eat anything at all and lost quite a bit of weight and the time I spent on the ward was a mix of trying to stay in my own bubble and being affected by other patients. I did get the orange cup and some other orange things including some clothes I had already bought. Vera brought in some orange 'Viscount biscuits' in the hope I would eat them but I never did. I was medicated once with Acuphase because I refused to turn the volume down on the CD player which Carmen had brought to the ward. Acuphase is a fast acting drug used to sedate and a drug that can sometimes be used as a punishment. I only saw it happen once when a patient was frog marched to his bed and injected simply because he told a nurse, "I am not fuckin' mad". Apparently it wasn't what he said but the manner in which he had said it that made it necessary to sedate him. The music I played was a mixture of old and new but there were messages in the music and not just for me, I would also sometimes use songs to express the way I felt. Henry put on one of my CD's one morning just as Carmen had walked onto the ward and the song by Del Shannon was 'Little Town Flirt' and I probably looked into that a little too much. I became very worried when I thought about the work I had done with SMA in that I thought I was tackling stigma but had actually set my self up as a target. I wasn't educating anybody just letting them know I had been diagnosed whereas if I had blended into my community the stigma wouldn't have affected me as much. I had put myself into the limelight and I had possibly angered those who had had me diagnosed in the first place. Throughout my time on P-1 I thought it was a massive experiment and that the patients had been 'planted' and there were cameras or listening devices everywhere. There were those thoughts and the other thoughts I have already mentioned plus a lot of ideas that I revisited from 1991. I kept my thoughts and ideas to myself most of the time and especially on the morning of the mental health tribunal. Of course by then my mode of thinking was much more conventional because the Larcagtil had been doing its job.

Harry put forward his case then my legal representative put forward mine and my main point was that I wasn't a danger to myself or anybody else. Margaret had some input too of course and sitting there in my wedding suit which now seemed at least one size too big I felt confident that I was going home. I was absolutely famished and was wondering whether Carmen had brought the cheese salad sandwiches I had asked for. Harry informed the panel that I thought there was a man travelling on the bus with a bomb in his bag. As it was only Carmen that I had mentioned that to I wondered just how and when he had gotten to know about it. "Yes and did she tell you he was Irish stew" I blurted out. "I mean too, he was Irish too" I said. There was a titter of laughter and Harry said, "He hasn't been eating either". Now Harry didn't expect that there would be even more amusement from that comment but there was. I won the appeal and afterwards Margaret told Carmen and me that the panel wished us well and that they said 'we make a lovely couple'. I had to sign something to say I was leaving the hospital against medical advice, because I had refused to stay as a voluntary patient when Harry had asked me to.

Chapter Ten: Royalty and a knighthood

Carmen and I were married on the 12th April and most of our family members and friends attended the wedding. Those that didn't attend were my eldest half brother George and his family, my sister Karla and her kids, two of Carmen's sisters and unfortunately Elaine, Carmen's mum, didn't come either. I felt sorry for Carmen because for their own reasons Elaine and two of Carmen's sisters had let her down on what was a very happy day for both of us. My friends from SMA and some of our neighbours were there and I met Carmen's Aunt and Uncle who I am pleased to say are still good friends today. On all of the wedding photos I looked very red faced as though maybe I had fallen asleep beneath a sun-bed but this was down to the Largactil. The hotel where we held the reception was a hotel called Royals and it was all paid for by American Express and so was our honeymoon. We spent a couple of days in Southport and apart from the occasion where the police phoned our hotel for Carmen to collect me it all went well. I had gone into the police station just across from the hotel and made allegations of police corruption in the Greater Manchester Police force, I also stated they were covering up child abuse. Our main honeymoon a few days later was spent in Paris and whilst there I kept my nose clean so to speak, I did however buy lots of orange things. I bought Carmen a designer orange dress and myself an orange coat, and as well as these purchases American Express also paid for our meals and presents for the kids. We did the trip down the Seine on a pleasure boat, we visited Notre Dame and the Louvre and in all I found Paris to be a wonderful city.

Back in Manchester at home I thought things were going along well I was now married and the New Labour theme of 'Things Can Only Get Better' rang true for us all. The trouble was rather than take the chlorpromazine regularly I was using it PRN and it became used by me less and less. I had remembered the worries about the tardive dyskinesia so I did have valid reasons for not taking it as often. I was sectioned on 1st May 1997 (polling day) this time I had destroyed the cylinder for the hot water in our home and I had also 'kidnapped' my son Ashley. Ashley had returned with Carmen from the local shops and I could see that my four year old had a black eye. When I asked Carmen about the shiner she seemed very blasé about it simply saying he wasn't looking where he was going.

Ashley and I were in a taxi on the outskirts of Moss Side when the driver's radio announced – 'A fare from South Manchester with a red haired adult and a little boy, the adult is not well, it is a police matter please radio in with your whereabouts'. "What should I do?" The driver said looking at me. I looked onto the backseat where Ashley was sleeping and told the driver to take us back to the house where he had collected us from. The police took me in a police van directly to Withington Hospital and Margaret followed us in her car, I was put back onto ward P-1.

I was on the ward for about four weeks and I lost my appeal against the section. I was thinking about all of my children including those I hadn't seen since they were babies. The morning after my admission the telly was on and Tony Blair, his wife and children were assembled for a photo-call outside number 10. Another patient made the comment that she couldn't believe his children were wearing 'Tory blue'. At the time I was really worried about the safety of Carmen and the kids and this was all mixed in with my other thoughts of what was happening. I remember I had been back on the ward about a week when a member of staff named Colin decided to read out loud from his newspaper, 'The Torygraph'. "Isn't that terrible, a man was in hospital when his wife and kids were all killed in a house fire" he said. I stood up and crossed the lounge to where he was sat and without hesitation punched him in the mouth. He stood and I could tell he wanted to hit me back so I stood back. "C'mon then you bastard what do you want me to do I can't just go home I am sectioned". Henry who was still a patient on the ward shouted, "Tony leave it he's a fuckin' Commando". It was the only time Henry had called me anything other than Billy. I was medicated and spent the next 24 hours chemically restrained on my bed. An older patient told me a few days later that I had done right as Colin was 'army trash', I wasn't so sure though. One thing that did happen after that incident was that at every opportunity I could do I would set off the fire alarms on ward P-1. When the firemen would arrive I would tell them who I was and to remember my name in case anything happens.

The then nursing staff of P-1 and indeed of the other psychiatric wards of today are made up of both qualified nurses and 'bank' or agency staff. Whether all or any of the bank staff have nursing qualifications I don't know and whether there is a vetting procedure for non qualified or agency staff I don't know either. The trouble was that it wasn't always easy to know who was and who wasn't a 'real nurse' and then there were student nurses. Some would actually identify or introduce themselves as students, as nurses or as support workers and some wouldn't. There were also some staff who objected to being asked by the patient and in my experience the objectors were usually just there to 'make up the numbers'. I am not saying it is easy for a hospital trust to staff a ward just that there didn't seem to be any monitoring or evaluation of good practice. I have never known visitors or inspectors independent of the trust (or the ward) come in and speak to patients about the care they are receiving. Now it may be that the job of ensuring that everything was done properly was up to the qualified psychiatric nurse in charge of the ward. Assuming that the person in charge has a professional approach themselves it still isn't easy for them to oversee all that happens on the ward. I am sure though that there must be rules about the ratio of qualified staff on a ward at any one time. Luckily the layout and the way P-1 was designed meant that there was usually at least one caring member of staff within sight or earshot. There are relationships and friendships amongst staff too and just like anyone else they are human and have prejudices of their own. So in that group, like in any group, there are good and bad or professional and unprofessional amongst them. It wasn't just about qualifications either because even though nursing is seen as a vocational thing there were some who in my opinion were just 'pulling a wage'. Qualified people who acted as security guards and there were people who would probably only ever qualify as a security guard and they thought they were nurses. It is this big thing about care versus control again, although I do accept that some patients may need to be restrained. What I cannot accept is the use of excessive force because to me it is assault by the back door so to speak. Then there is outright assault and what is more difficult to prove is when there are two members of staff and each saying that you attacked them.

I would see Colin arrive for his shift with a cut and bruised lip and as the medication started to have an affect on me I decided I owed him an apology. I had stopped setting the fire alarms off because I was informed that the hospital was charged each time the fire brigade was called out. I had tried to escape from the ward a few times too and on two occasions the electronic door had to be repaired. A nurse told me I was in danger of bankrupting the trust at the rate I was going so I stopped doing it. Colin and another member of staff named Matt were glaring at me on one occasion and it made me very nervous. A little later I went into the room next to the lounge it was the room that housed the pool table and had the door leading to the Garden. I waited there for Colin to come back inside as he was smoking in the Garden, it was about 9pm. When he entered the room and locked the outside door I put my hand out and told him I wasn't thinking clearly and that I was very sorry for hitting him. He shook my hand but as he did so he switched the lights out with his other hand then he kneed me in my balls and I went down. He was on top of me and hit me in my head before he shouted for help and he told the staff who arrived that I had attacked him again. I was chemically restrained again and spent another few days on my bed and my visitors were turned away from the ward. It was my second week on the ward and essentially my thinking was a lot better. I had everything neatly filed back into the kisamo box, I was eating regular food again and I was expecting to be moved to another ward. I was sat listening to the end of a Miles Davies CD one evening and I got up to change the disc for some Woody Guthrie. As I stood up Matt one of the staff pulled across the curtain on the side of the room where my CD player was. I expected him to cross the room and pull the other curtain so that they met in the middle but he never. I was just trying to find the Guthrie disc when I actually saw stars, stars because Matt had just punched me in the side of my head. He caught the top of my ear and the temple of the right side of my head. This was witnessed by another patient but not by the person on ward P-10. Like everyone else on P-1 Matt knew somebody was watching from the other ward hence the curtain and hence Colin switching the light out. Matt was on top of me pushing my head down and shouting for help, he said I had 'attacked him' and I was duly medicated. The other patient was scared out of his wits and by the time I had recovered from the Acuphase he had been discharged to the street. Apparently he didn't have a mental illness and was homeless and he confessed that fact to staff whilst I slept. Basically both of the incidents, firstly with Colin and then with Matt were a case of my word against theirs. In actual fact though it was a case of two friends exacting revenge for something I actually regretted doing.

I was eventually discharged from hospital and the Depixol injections were reinstated but not before I had delusions of grandeur, I was the 'prince of orange' I was royalty! Perhaps it was the feeling of being important because all of the things that were being done were all for my benefit. Or perhaps it was also everything else; my grandfather had a German 'royal' surname, the orange viscount biscuits, the cigarette packets or the hotel where I was married. Then there was the solicitor telling me, 'you'll be treated like royalty if you do go to prison'. "I have royal blood in me and this is what the whole thing is about, I am the prince of orange" I said to Harry. I explained to him about Henry calling me Billy and about the patients on Ward P-5 and 6 saying I was a German. "You do know that I am a psychiatrist?" he said. "Yes I know but that's not your fault don't worry I will look after you". As I say I was discharged to Harry's outpatient clinic and I only saw him again once because yet again I was going to be given a new psychiatrist.

The court case regarding my assault on Dawson was in the June of 1997 and Carmen, Vera and Andy supported me on the day of sentencing. The judge told me I had actually only escaped a custodial sentence by the skin of my teeth. He was particularly keen to emphasise that people just cannot take the law into their own hands. I was given a two year sentence which was suspended for two years so in effect if I kept my nose clean it was all over with. Dawson pleaded not guilty in the August and for obvious reasons I didn't attend his trial. I did however support Lorna on the day of her testimony when she gave evidence from a different part of the court buildings via a video link. After she had finished and came back into the waiting area she told me that I had been described as unpredictable, volatile, aggressive and extremely violent. Dawson was using the assault by me on him as part of his defence, implying Lorna had no option but to say he abused her because she was afraid of me. It also came to light that Karla my sister gave evidence for Dawson stating she had no doubts and that he definitely hadn't abused Lorna. That was the reason nobody had heard from her the past few months as she knew she was going to be a witness for her husband. It wasn't mentioned in court that on one occasion Karla had hidden under the bed where Lorna was sleeping because of something her own daughter had said to her about her own father. There was also the red herring that whilst the abuse was taking place Dawson was involved with Lorna's mum Anne as it was before she had met her husband. Dawson walked away from court free as a bird and Karla was ostracised by the whole family. I have heard from different family members little bits of information of the abuse of Lorna. It had started as inappropriate kissing at bedtime and progressed into sexual abuse and Lorna herself has mentioned some things to me. I try not to think about it because it hurts me and I try not to think about the people in my family that had helped him get away with it.

Margaret had spoken to Harry about my American Express debt which was in excess of £8,000 and one of the last things Harry did for me was write to the company. The letter I received from them thanked me for using American Express and said I owed them nothing and if I hadn't already I should cut up the card. The letter was addressed to 'Sir Anthony Scallly' I didn't look anything into that too much as I assumed it was a typographical error of some kind. I remained well for the next six years and was seeing different doctors on each outpatient appointment for the next two and a half years. I complained to the Hospital trust about lack of continuity and stability with the many different psychiatrists I was seeing. I was told that once the trust had transferred over to a new site in South Manchester I would be assigned a permanent doctor.

The Rev Sarah fellows talked me into volunteering to work in the church youth club and she also talked me into editing the church magazine. Carmen and I often joked about Sarah and the way she got people to 'volunteer' in that she was a 'Columbo' type of character. One way or another she was bound to wear you down even if it was just by sheer persistence. However I did enjoy doing the magazine and being a part of the youth group. I befriended a few of the young people and through one of the members I met Tina who 'self harmed', she was 18 years old at the time. Carmen decided that she wanted to get into the health profession and joined a college and an access into health course. Our marriage on the whole was a good one and not unlike any other we had our moments, there was sometimes bickering and sometimes there were full blown arguments. The happier times far outweighed the argumentative ones though and in all our time together I only ever directly accused Carmen of cheating twice. I had thought that she was on other occasions but I never said anything and the arguments were quite often relating to something else. We are good parents and so our tiffs and rows would never affect the children as we just didn't do it whilst they were around. As I say it wasn't anything major and not often. It was usually around issues of my sleeping or the fact that I hadn't quit smoking as I often promised I would. I spent the happiest years of my life with Carmen and the children and wouldn't change that experience for anything.

Brian was still seeing the children every so often although from time to time he would disappear for months on end and Carmen would say that he was probably locked up. The children started to resent going to church so we never forced them into going and I myself still avoided the services. As I have said though I did have an active role as a church volunteer and was also an out-of-hours key holder for times when the alarm went off. I also sat on the management committee of a local children's project again at Sarah's 'invitation'. Carmen, the children and I had some fantastic holidays each year and we all explored and discovered Cornwall and Devon together. I was getting better with my reading and watching the telly and for two full football seasons I watched the premiership winners and losers. Margaret Warburton eventually did retire and my new social worker was Claire and I liked her immediately. I had lost contact with most of my SMA friends when the agency was wound up in 1998, I say most of them but Tom Kendall and Ollie Richards kept in touch. Carmen did a year at Liverpool University on a radiotherapy degree course but after it became impossible for her to commute she dropped out. Carmen was out one day when I got a visit from Greater Manchester police and the two officers were working on 'operation Cleopatra'. They wanted to know of my experiences in care homes during the 70s and 80s and I told them it was a can of worms I would rather not open. They had gotten my details from Social Services and were fully aware of my mental health issues. I explained that I was very ill the last time I had thoughts about my experiences of the time I spent in care. They left me with two cards one a contact for the operation and another was a free counselling service. I never contacted either but did discuss the matter with the project worker from the local children's project. Although she never gave advice as such I decided that Burnett if he was still alive didn't pose a risk to other children as he would be too old to be still working with them.

Lorna came to live with us for a short time when her mum separated from her step father. Only a short time because it never really worked out and it was a stressful time for all concerned not least Lorna herself. It ended with both Lorna and Carmen putting me in the position where I had to choose between them. However as I have said previously I also had Ashley to consider. Lorna maintains to this day that Carmen never actually ever wanted her living with us and says Carmen went out of her way to set her up in a way that meant it was never going to work out. I became more like a Henry Kissinger between them rather than a father or a husband. Lorna ended up back with Vera in the end but not before spending two nights in hospital because she had swallowed a dozen strong painkillers.

Carmen decided to go into general adult nursing and qualified in 2002 and it was at that time Carmen told me she wanted to move. Carmen said that she wanted us to live and for her to work in Cornwall but she later changed her mind. At first she was offered a job at Truro Royal Hospital and it was the accommodation that was proving difficult then as I say she suddenly changed her mind. The whole idea was dropped when she took up a post at Wythenshawe General Hospital. Patsy and Pete separated and Pete and I haven't seen eye to eye since then because of the way I felt he had let Patsy and himself down. They were divorced eighteen months after separating and Patsy kept the smaller of their two shops open by selling second hand goods. However by the time he was divorced Pete had lost the bigger shop and was looking for work, which goes to show how much of a positive influence Patsy had been for him.

I took care of the house and the children whilst Carmen did her nursing during the week and at weekend we did it between us. Now the South Manchester Psychiatric service had all been transferred to a purpose built unit at Wythenshawe hospital. It was called Laureate House and the wards were named after famous authors like the Bronte's or poets like Blake. My new psychiatrist was Dr. Steve Newall and I liked him straightaway, so much so that after our initial meeting I wrote and told him so. I learnt more about the life of Tina in that she had herself suffered abuse as a child and now she seemed to have quite a reckless approach to life. She never did drugs in my presence but I became aware that she was getting 'stuff' locally and sometimes when I saw her she was under the influence. There would be fresh cuts on her arms and once she commented to me that 'brown' (heroin) helps her to forget. The Rev Sarah fellows left the parish and a younger minister named Kathy replaced her. Claire would visit us from time to time and like Margaret it wasn't an officious relationship she had with me. My sleeping in the afternoon became a fixed routine in that once the housework was done I would sleep until the kids got home from school. Carmen and I decided we would buy our house off the council and we applied for a mortgage. We bought a Renault scenic people carrier it was a larger, newer and more practical vehicle. At weekends and when the children were on holidays from school I would take them swimming and weather permitting we would do some outdoor activities.

Whether it was daytrips to the seaside, going out locally to Styal woods or a tour of Quarry Bank Mill we always tried to do something. Carmen and I hardly ever went out together or socialised although Carmen had one friend who she would sometimes go out with in the evenings. On our birthdays Carmen and I would always go to the same restaurant for a meal.

Tina would help me with the photocopying and the stapling of the church magazine sometimes but there were times where nobody saw her for weeks on end. Carmen started doing bank (or agency) work on some of the general wards at Wythenshawe hospital and that took her away at weekends. She started going to work earlier and coming home later on weekdays and the shifts at weekend varied from week to week. We didn't really need the money so I did become a little concerned, then the text messages to her phone and the emails started to arrive. I did truly want to stick everything into the kisamo box just as I had done throughout our marriage with various things. Things and people, and things that people had said I had all sorts in that box. The trouble was Dr. Newall and I were trying me out on an atypical oral medication called Olanzapine at around that time.

It was the 5th November 2003 I was sat in our bedroom, the children were watching the telly and I could hear them laughing downstairs. I had become more and more worried about my relationship with Carmen as we were drifting apart at a rapid rate. She started to suggest that I wasn't the person she had met all those years ago which was true I guess in the physical sense but essentially I was still me. There had become no such thing as affection unless you count the quick peck on the cheek that replaced the once passionate kisses. There had been phone calls to our house phone and it was a man who always asked for another person by name. It didn't matter how many times he was told there was nobody by that name the calls had persisted over the past few months. I was sat up in my room convinced it was some sort of code between Carmen and her lover, yes I thought she was seeing somebody again. As I say sitting there I had these thoughts and I was becoming more distressed and filled with rage whilst thinking about it. I had thoughts of taking every door off every hinge and smashing every window in the house. I was thinking of destroying every stick of furniture but I couldn't what about the kids. As soon as Carmen got home I left the house but I didn't know where I was going to go and then decided I needed to get some help. I went around to church and let myself in and from the vestry I telephoned the mental health liaison team for South Manchester.

It was a friend from the old Day Hospital who took my call a nurse named Sue Blakeley. "Tony, make your way to the casualty at Wythenshawe hospital get a taxi if you need to and I will be waiting here for you" she said.

Because I am still a patient under Laureate House this is another portion of the book where I need to be careful. Laureate House is the hospital unit where I would go tomorrow if I became unwell so I mustn't really be too critical and need to be succinct at this stage.

Sue was there waiting for me and she made sure that I had cigarettes and money to see me through what I thought was going to be a brief admission for assessment. Although I presented myself at the hospital I was actually sectioned first with a section 2 and then a few days later with a section 3. Of course I lodged an appeal and sought legal representation from a list of local solicitors that a nurse gave to me. I wasn't allowed off Bronte ward and was worried that I would be in hospital over the Christmas period. I told Vera I didn't want any visitors as I didn't really want her making the long journey across Manchester each day. It was a surreal experience at first in that one of the first patients I had met on Bronte ward was Henry Vance. Then there were a couple of the other patients that worried me greatly and I knew them from the 80s. One of them belonged in the kisamo box and I actually put him there but he escaped a week later.

Just to clarify the kisamo box is just a separation in my head where things or incidents go that need to be dealt with separately. I did have a lot in there around issues relating to my wife but on this occasion the individual as far as I knew didn't know her. He belonged in the box because of an incident twenty years ago which was before I knew Carmen.

Carmen visited me on one occasion and she was wearing new clothes which she had bought 'to cheer herself up'. I directly accused her of cheating on me and that it was probably with somebody who actually worked at Wythenshawe Hospital. "Tony you're not well I am not seeing anybody" she said. "I have been here nine days if I am not well then where is my get well card?" I said. "It's almost Christmas and you know that" she told me. "Fair enough where is my Christmas card I sent you one and I have had get well cards from other people". I knew at that very moment from the look on her face I had lost her and she herself was lost for words. She had bought clothes to cheer herself up and couldn't find a few pence for a Christmas card I could hardly believe my ears.

I lost the appeal because a trickcylist told the panel that I had told him I was 'tormented by the voices'. I told them it was an outright lie and the one thing I had clung on to all these years is the fact that I didn't hear voices. It was plainly an attempt to neatly parcel me up in that psychiatric box marked 'schizophrenia'. "You were upset and extremely tearful" the trickcylist said in his defence. "I was thinking about my children and my wife" I told them all. As I say I lost the appeal and was extremely worried as it looked like I would have to accept treatment or be on the ward a long time. It meant going back onto the depot injection but I truly felt that the Olanzapine was working and that I had real issues around my wife and her disloyalty. Being the typical stubborn stupid fool that I am I decided that I would no longer agree to take the Olanzapine. I looked at Claire and said, "Right they won't let me out of here so it's going to take more than the British Army to get me out".

As you can imagine stopping the Olanzapine wasn't really my shrewdest move as I began to lose insight. An elderly patient died in her sleep whilst I was on Bronte ward and it affected me a great deal. I didn't know her personally but on one occasion I could see she was frightened by the way another patient was acting in that he was doing practice karate kicks or kung fu in the lounge. Then there were the Bombings in Turkey that I heard about from the TV on the ward. The vending machine on the ward had a chocolate 'Turkish Delight' and the code to press if you wanted it was C4 which as you may be aware is plastic explosive. It was as if everything happening globally was centred on this psychiatric ward. I actually removed the TV aerial and threw it out of the window but it was eventually retrieved and put back. Another time a character from a soap opera only had one eyebrow and when I asked the other patient watching why she said, "Oh that's just because he is mad, that's bomb 'ed". I asked her why they called him 'bomb head' and again she said, "Because he is mad, they call him bomb 'ed". I sometimes feel as though a bomb has gone off in my head so I decided to shave both my own eyebrows off. When I got back into the lounge eyebrowless, the news item on telly was to do with Edinburgh University. I began to panic, what have I done, a bomb is now going to go off in Edinburgh that's what 'bomb 'ed' means. The 'ed' could actually be referring to education or the university this is all my fault! I had well and truly lost the plot and had to be medicated, I slipped in and out of consciousness over the next 12 hours. I woke up on the secure Blake ward where I eventually agreed to go back onto the depot injection. I was discharged from Blake ward in time to spend Christmas at home.

I have to state that in every hospital admission I have had as well as encountering the nursing staff I have already spoken about I met lots of dedicated, caring and professional nursing staff. In fact the 'good nurses' (including bank staff) and doctors make up the majority of Manchester's mental health service. It's this whole thing of there being minorities in any large group of people whether that is amongst the medical staff or the patients.

Carmen and I separated shortly after our 7th wedding anniversary in the April of 2004 and we were divorced 12 months later. It was all entirely her decision but I went along with it because I knew she was unhappy. I signed all of the mortgage papers over to Carmen and I was offered a two bedroom flat locally by the city council. I couldn't make her be in love with me the way I was with her and the last thing I wanted was for her to be unhappy. I didn't see it as a cliché because nobody had ever said it to me before but Carmen stated that she did love me but was not in love with me. I moved into the flat which is five minutes walk away from where I used to live, and I now see Ashley and my step children regularly. I have also re-established contact with all of my other children including one daughter I knew nothing about. This is because when I separated from her mum I didn't know her mother was pregnant at that time. Within a period of twelve months I moved house was divorced and I suffered bereavement so it isn't surprising I have had a brief hospital admission since then. My friend Tina was found lying dead at her grandmother's house and she had an empty syringe by her side. I also heard recently through the grapevine that my friend from school Jay died in very similar circumstances.

For the sake of Ashley and the other children Carmen and I are still on talking terms but it isn't the same in the post divorce milieu. Ashley just like my other children is excelling at school and in a conversation recently he told me he may become a psychiatrist. There was a time he would have been grounded for such a remark but I can't think of a more worthwhile career if that is what he wants to do.

Nobody can pinpoint why my mind began working the way it does and this book isn't an attempt for me to do that. The research into schizophrenia is still ongoing and so is the debate that Dr. Declan told me about fifteen years ago. The genetic argument hasn't been entirely proven, not even with the studies involving identical twins. Schizophrenia can run in families but religion runs in families too and yet we don't assume that there is a Catholic gene or a Presbyterian gene. The high prevalence of schizophrenia in inner cities or urban areas and cannabis playing a role only adds to the mystery. Some say that it is all about being predisposed or susceptible to an episode of illness and it is then that genetics and the use of street drugs come into play. Others say it's all about childhood trauma or the way the developing brain deals with life events. There's research involving the infant brain, adolescent or teenage brain, and some scientists are going as far back as the foetal or embryonic brain cells. I mentioned the GIGO theory to my daughter Lorna and she told me that the brain may not show physical scars but she believes it does become scarred. The mind, psyche or 'the soul' isn't visible so cannot easily be mended. If you bang nails into a fence, even if you remove the nails later, the holes are still there.

I certainly don't blame any one person for me becoming ill and although I complain about being diagnosed I know there are some who just don't deserve treatment. What I mean is there are some places in the world where either poverty or war, or both means that people are just left to get on with it. My current support worker pointed out that by writing this book it may put me back into the limelight and may adversely affect my health. It is a good point but there is nothing you have read here that is going to shake the world. I just felt it was something that needed to be written and it needs to be out there. There is nothing more I can do for the mental health service user/survivor movement, but what I will say, is no matter what your diagnosis is you have the right to write.

Everything in this book is based on my own experience and unless otherwise stated all of the opinions are my own.

Printed in the United Kingdom by
Lightning Source UK Ltd., Milton Keynes
137396UK00001B/76/A